New Year, New You

Natalia Krasnyanskaya
& the Editors of Top.me

ISBN: 1503272621
ISBN-13: 978-1503272620

New Year, New You

CONTENTS

New Year, New You

INTRODUCTION

Congratulations! You took action by buying this book. This year is going to be the year you will take control over your body.

With my guide, you will learn which exercises are the most effective and which exercises to avoid.

The workouts, divided into easy monthly units, are designed not just to help you lose weight but also to shape and tone your body.

Between the months, I have included helpful and practical articles on how to boost your metabolism, which cardio is the most effective, and what you need to include in your diet. I'll even show you how to keep up today's motivation – for the whole year!

You will love your new image in the mirror. Welcome the new healthy, fit you!

Natalia Krasnyanskaya
Editor in Chief, top.me

1 FIVE REASONS TO GET IN SHAPE THIS YEAR

Did you know the number one health risk has shifted worldwide from starvation to obesity?

In 1950, the number of starving individuals on Earth was estimated to be around 700 million. At the time, obesity affected approximately 100 million people around the globe, primarily in rich countries.

These statistics have changed dramatically over the past six decades. The rate of "extreme obesity" (people with a BMI above 40) rose by 350 percent over the past few years alone in the US.

The sad fact is more people collectively across the world are now suffering from being fat than from not having enough food to eat. One estimate puts the number of obese at 1 billion compared to 800 million people who are underfed.

In the United States, obesity has become a huge problem. According to research published in 2013 by the University of Colorado at Boulder[1], one in five American deaths is now associated with obesity.

---

[1]Ryan K. Masters, et.al. The Impact of Obesity on US Mortality Levels: The Importance of Age and Cohort Factors in Population Estimates. American Journal of Public Health: October 2013, Vol. 103, No. 10, pp. 1895-1901.

The western diet consists of many unhealthy and processed foods that lack nutrients and this seems to have a major influence on energy levels and motivation.

I am a firm believer that being in good shape has such a positive impact on your whole life. Let's take a look at the five reasons you should get in shape now.

It Will Make You Happy

You probably don't need any other reason but this one. Exercising helps to release endorphins in your brain, which release the "feel good" emotion. Working out will help you become a happier person. Researchers at the Penn State Social Science Research Institute recently concluded[2] that "people who are more physically active have more pleasant-activated feelings than people who are less active."

Not to mention that if you are in shape and you feel like you look good physically, this has major impacts on happiness. A review of 15 clinical studies[3] found a clear link between obesity and depression. Yet another great reason you should get in shape.

It Will Prevent Serious Health Problems

Let's be honest here – who wants to actually be obese? I would guess very few people do. Obesity is the result of a lifestyle, not a decision. People suffer from obesity all around the world, and there is a long list of health problems associated with obesity, like hypertension, diabetes, congestive heart failure, high blood pressure, and stroke. If you are an obese

---

[2] http://www.hhd.psu.edu/news/2012/Physical-Activity-Feelings.html

[33] Luppino FS, de Wit LM, Bouvy PF, et al. Overweight, Obesity, and Depression: A Systematic Review and Meta-analysis of Longitudinal Studies. Arch Gen Psychiatry. 2010;67(3):220-229.

person, you are much more likely to suffer from one of these serious illnesses.

It Will Increase Your Confidence

When you look your best, you will feel your best and act your best. Getting in great shape is certain to boost your confidence, which will have a positive catalyst in all areas of your life. You will be much more confident in the dating scene as well when you are in great shape. Many overweight people lack confidence due to their physical appearance. People who take pride in their body's and their appearance will likely take pride in all facets of life.

It Will Increase Your Energy Levels

Exercising to increase your energy levels is a funny concept. Most people think that after you exercise you are going to be tired and exhausted all day but the opposite actually happens. People who exercise regularly have higher energy levels.

If you are looking for a great all day energy boost, try exercising in the morning before you go to work.

Exercise is Fun and Enjoyable

Exercise can be a really fun and enjoyable experience. People who don't exercise have a bad perception that working out and being in shape is a giant chore. This is not true at all! Nobody said that getting in shape had to be boring. You can choose a multitude of activities such as playing your favorite sport, lifting weights, running, jumping rope, sprinting, and even dancing! Pick a few of your favorite ones and you are on your way.

Before Exercising

Always have water with you to prevent dehydration. Remember to stretch at the beginning of each workout and when you are done. In case of feeling bad or uncomfortable, stop exercising.

2 WHAT IS HIGH INTENSITY INTERVAL TRAINING

Unless you've been living in cave without an internet connection for the past 15 years, you will have heard have heard about High Intensity Interval Training (HIIT). While the 1980s was all about Aerobics, HIIT has occupied the top of the fitness mountain since the late 90s.

The Benefits of HIIT

Typical low intensity cardio, such as running, is not effective for weight loss. In fact, a study performed by researchers at the Arizona State University in Phoenix, Arizona,[4] came to a surprising finding. They recruited 81 overweight women to run on the treadmill three times a week,

---

[4] http://journals.lww.com/nsca-jscr/Abstract/publishahead/Predictors_of_fat_mass_changes_in_response_to.97161.aspx

7

30 minutes each time. The women did not need to change their diet. What do you think the result was? A whopping 70 percent of the women actually gained weight! And the weight gain consisted of fat tissue, not muscle.

So what is HIIT and why is it better than low intensity cardio? In short, HIIT offers an exercise approach that improves cardiovascular health, extends life expectancy, and burns fat while preserving muscle mass while by training with high intensity, for short bursts of time.

Aerobic Effects

The Aerobics craze of the 1980s had people jogging and attending group gym classes with tight leotards and head bands. It was a thought that a minimum of 20-40 minutes a week of aerobic exercise was needed to maintain a good level of health. While this isn't incorrect, it is only half the story.

The measure of aerobic capacity is something called the VO2max. Put simply, this is the maximum of oxygen the lungs can transport to working muscles during exercise. Studies into HIIT show conclusively that exercisers performing intense intervals for a relatively short duration achieve the same or better improvements in VO2max than those performing long sessions of steady state cardio.

Metabolic Effects

In terms of metabolism, intensity matters. HIIT elevates metabolism (and therefore fat burning capacity) because it is such a dramatic, positive stress on the body. The body spends the hours following exercise recovering. Muscles are in oxygen debt so breathing is elevated. This excess post-exercise oxygen consumption (EPOC or 'after burn effect') can improve fat burning ability for as much as 24 hours after.

Other benefits to the metabolism include:

Lactate removal — HIIT is by nature anaerobic, that is, exercise depletes muscle energy faster than oxygen can be transported to replenish them. In the absence of oxygen, muscles cannot regenerate ATP (adenosine triphosphate, the useable form of energy to muscles) so waste products (lactate) accumulate causing fatigue. HIIT will improve your muscles' ability to metabolize lactate and therefore improves recovery. [5]

Insulin sensitivity — Researchers have also found that HIIT can also improve the body's ability to process glucose,[6] meaning muscle energy stores (glycogen) are more readily replenished and blood sugar spikes even out quickly. The opposite of such efficient insulin production — insulin resistance — is the condition known as diabetes. The Gibala study (details below) showed a 35% increase in insulin sensitivity over 2 weeks for 7 sedentary adult subjects.

Scientific Studies Supporting HIIT

Thankfully, we have numerous studies we can point to that show how HIIT is in many cases superior to traditional steady state cardio (e.g. jogging at a manageable pace).

The Tabata Study

Probably the most famous scheme HIIT workout comes from the famous study performed in 1996 by Izumi Tabata.[7] Not only was this a ground-breaking study in exercise science, the Tabata study is appealing because one round of intervals takes a mere 4 minutes. Something so stunningly simple and time efficient that could produce great improvements in cardiovascular fitness and overall health was destined for stardom.

Tabata compared the results from a group of speed skaters performing steady state cardio at 70% VO2max, 5 times per week with a group doing a specific set of interval training at

---

[5] http://www.ncbi.nlm.nih.gov/pubmed/19088769

[6] http://www.ncbi.nlm.nih.gov/pmc/articles/PMC2640399/

[7] http://www.ncbi.nlm.nih.gov/pubmed/8897392

170% VO2max just 3 times per week. Tabata found that not only did the group performing HIIT achieve greater gains in VO2max, they also made gains in anaerobic capacity that the control group did not.

The Gibala Study

Professor Martin Gibala of McMaster University conducted another famous study in 2009[8]. This study employed up to 12 rounds of longer intervals at a lower intensity than Tabata, with rest periods of 75 seconds. Just like the Tabata, Gibala et al found that the exercisers employing the HIIT approach 3 times per week made similar gains to those putting in 5 days a week of steady state cardio (50–70% VO2max). R

Other recent studies include:
• The Effect of In-season, High-Intensity Interval Training in Soccer Players[9]
• High-Intensity Interval Training: Applications for General Fitness Training [10]

Different Types of HIIT

HIIT comes in many forms and can be adapted to suit anyone's fitness level, activity preference and lifestyle.

Tabata Intervals

A Tabata workout lasts just 4 minutes and includes a simple workout to rest ratio. For every 20 seconds of exercise you rest a mere 10 seconds. Perform this style workout for 8 rounds

---

[8] http://jp.physoc.org/content/575/3/901.abstract

[9]

http://www.fmh.utl.pt/agon/cpfmh/docs/documentos/recursos/112/DupontSoccerIntTraining.pdf

[10] http://www.lookgreatnaked.com/articles/high_intensity_interval_training.pdf

and you're done. This really is exercise minimalism at its finest.

There is nothing stopping you from doing more rounds if you are really fit. Most people find the 4-minute workout three times a week to be sufficient to significantly improve cardiovascular health.

Gibala Intervals

In this regimen of interval training, complete 8-12 rounds of 60 second intervals at 95% VO2max, followed by 75 seconds of rest.

Suggested Equipment for HIIT

The only equipment you'll need is a good timer. You can buy special timers that you can program specific intervals into or simply use your smartphone. You will need these because chances are you won't be able to concentrate on counting when your body's main concern is getting enough oxygen!

A good, cheap interval timer is the Gymboss timer, but there are many others out there.

Here are a couple of good HIIT apps for iPhone and Android:
iPhone apps:
• Fast Exercise
• Interval Timer for HIIT Training and Workouts
Android apps:
• HIIT interval training timer
• A HIIT Interval Timer

Dangers of HIIT

The biggest danger with any intense exercise program is overtraining. It is tempting to think that because HIIT workouts are short compared to other forms of conditioning, more workload can be safely added to the regimen.

Trainers call this overreaching, which over time can lead to overtraining as fatigue builds up and the body fails to cope properly.

The important point here is "stimulate don't annihilate". Make sure you are fully recovered between workouts — don't multiply your fatigue by pushing yourself again too soon.

Frequent Questions

What time of the day is best to do HIIT?

The answer to this one is by no means definite. Some swear by morning workouts, while others prefer the afternoon or evening. There is one problem with morning workouts: make sure you don't do your HIIT workout on an empty stomach. Fat is burned hours after your workout. If you work out on an empty stomach, your body will prioritize muscle loss before fat loss.

What's the ideal intensity?

High. Most of the time you should be working at as fast as you can with good form. However, protocols with longer interval durations (30s plus) might require lower intensities. If you think of exercise intensity in terms of a 1-10 scale, HIIT efforts should be from 7-10.

What's the ideal length of a workout?

The ideal length depends on your fitness level, age and a number of health factors. Generally, you should be exhausted after a workout. This could be four minutes for one person and 20 minutes for the next. The sweet spot for most exercisers is 10-15 minutes.

Is HIIT safe?

That depends. Because this form of exercise elevates the heart rate to high levels make sure you get the okay from your physician before embarking on any HIIT regimen. HIIT is good for most people but there are always risks and some people will not be suited to such intense activity so make sure you get checked out first.

Can I do HIIT and Strength Training on the same day?

Absolutely, but do your strength training first. HIIT actually serves as a great finishing workout and helps promote circulation to your muscles, aiding in recovery. The best part is that interval training can be done in a very short period of time so you're not compromising your resistance training with an extended cardio workout.

Top.me

3 NUTRITION – THE BASICS

Physical exercise needs to be accompanied by a nutritious, healthy, balanced diet for the best results.

There are pages and pages of advice available in books and online, but the basic rules are:

- eat from each of the food groups;
- calculate your caloric intake and how much you burn, then eat at a caloric deficit;
- exercise.

It's not as overwhelming as it might first seem, so don't panic! Add supplements to your daily regimen to boost vitamins and minerals, and be sensible about your choices. Everything is fine in moderation. It is important not to let your food and nutrition dictate your life, but understand some basics to educate yourself and fuel your body effectively.

What Is a Balanced Diet?

So, the major premise is that a balanced diet is necessary, but what exactly does a balanced diet include?

Proteins

These are essential to your body, especially muscles. Protein is made up of various amino acids and builds lean muscle tissue. It is essential for repair and recovery of muscles after a workout and the intake should be increased when increasing physical activity. Sources of protein include eggs, lean red meat, and seafood. If you have a strenuous workout planned, eat some good meat, fish or eggs before and after. Did you know that in your diet you should aim for about 1 gram of protein for each pound of body weight?

Carbohydrates

Carbs are the fuel that runs the body. Modern society tends to view carbs as bad for the body, when in fact the ability to endure workouts would be made almost impossible without carbohydrates, which slowly release energy. Many diets tell you to cut out carbs altogether, but this has been proven only to have short-term results. No "anti-carb" diet will last the length of time; it's perfect for the beach body you're after for next month, but not a healthy lifestyle longer term. Over-consumption of carbohydrates store as fat, so there is some truth in the fact that they should be eaten in moderation, especially on less active days. The reason for this is that carbohydrates are not stored in body tissue, but by your liver and blood in limited amounts. The more you exercise the more carbs you need. The myth that carbohydrates are bad for you stems from refined carbs and sugars that send blood sugar levels soaring. Good, or "healthy," carbs come from whole fruits, whole vegetables and whole grains. These slowly release the energy you need to be active all day and spiking blood sugar levels.

Fats

When people see the word fat, they think of the artery-clogging, evil component that ruins bodies. But like carbs, fats are not all bad for you. We need fats in our diet. "Good" fats, such as Omega-3, are central for bodily functions such as metabolism, brain power, and the immune system. The problem with fats occurs when consuming too many saturated fat (such as high-fat dairy) and trans fats (found in sweets). Good nutrition needs a little common sense. Nothing comes easy, but if you learn to pick foods from different groups and keep meals varied, you should develop good habits that you can hold on to for years to come. Sensible eating means avoiding fast food and soda as well as cutting down on alcohol intake. Here are some tips for picking the best fats:

- Choose meat that is from a less fatty cut.
- Eat fatty fish such as salmon.
- Remove poultry skin.
- Choose all-natural, non-roasted, non-salted nuts.
- Use low-fat dairy when possible.

Did you know that the daily recommended intake of calories is 2,500 kcal for a man and 2,000 kcal for a woman?

Water

Water is absolutely crucial for your body. It is recommended to hydrate the body with lots of water (around 8 glasses a day), before, during, and after a workout. In fact, sometimes when you feel hungry, you're not hungry at all but actually dehydrated. A glass of water will fix the feeling without you needing any food.

Vitamins and Minerals

Most vitamins and minerals are found in a balanced diet. On packets of supplements the RDA (recommended daily allowance) is given, but this is the minimum amount needed per day. There is no harm in boosting certain vitamins and minerals, particularly if you omit certain foods from your diet. Fish oil capsules are a good starting point, as well as Vitamin D for those receiving less sunshine and Creatine for muscle-building and strength. If you are a vegetarian, this is a perfectly health way of living, however excluding meat or animal products from your diet should be replaced with certain vitamins, particular Vitamin B12, Iron, and Calcium to avoid any deficiencies.

Women's nutritional advice is similar to men's, but a woman should aim to include more iron in their diet, as well as Vitamin D, calcium, and folic acid for those thinking of having a child.

Generally, certain foods worth introducing to a good diet include:

- Avocado
- Cottage cheese
- Salmon
- Kidney beans
- Chick peas
- Walnuts

When choosing meat, pick lean cuts. Opt for whole wheat bread and pasta and skimmed milk. Tea and coffee are fine in moderation, as is the odd glass of wine, but the milk used in your cup of tea or coffee and the alcohol does add towards your daily calorie intake. Just be mindful of that!

The best healthy ways to cook are to steam or boil, bake, grill, or eat raw (vegetables). If oil is necessary, such as for stir frying, use Extra Virgin Olive Oil.

Cooking your own food from scratch ensures that you know what you are putting into your mouth. So get your apron on and the utensils out of the cupboard, invest in a good cook book and experiment. Better still, why not grow some fruits and vegetables in your garden? This could be your new hobby, and how great would your new dinner guests feel knowing they were eating home-grown, healthy food?

Every person is different and if you're unsure about what your personal calorie intake should be, there are a number of guides online that help calculate your weight/height, your exercise intensity and lifestyle. Some advice states that eating smaller portions, more regularly (5 times a day instead of 3), helps speed up your metabolism and help with blood sugar levels and the same goes for not eating straight before bed.

The most important point to clarify is that under-eating is as bad as over-eating. Starving the body from the calories and nutrients it needs is detrimental to its development and will not cause healthy weight loss. When you deny your body food, not only do you begin to burn muscle, but the metabolism does not function as quickly. As soon as you resume with eating, the body clings on to each meal as if it were its last, storing fat. Kick-starting your metabolism with breakfast and eating throughout the day will not only keep your body functioning at its optimum levels, but will help you feel energized for exercise. As a bonus, it will improve your skin, hair, nails, teeth, and overall mood and energy levels. Not a bad trade-off for a little extra time planning in the supermarket, is it?

Top.me

20

4 JANUARY

The New Year is here and your fitness resolutions are fresh in your mind. Not to mention that most of us have some holiday pounds to shed.

January's program is designed to kick-start your new year with a High Interval Training program using a mix of treadmill, weight, and functional fitness.

For most of us, it is too cold outside to take our regular training outdoors. Here are three workouts to rotate weekly as well as a tip on to make your driveway shoveling a workout.

As you have read before, HIIT workouts are characterized by short, intense bursts of exercise followed by short rest. These workouts include running and weightlifting so you will need to have access to a treadmill, a medicine ball, and some free weights.

Tip of the Month: Snow Shoveling

While most people try to avoid shoveling the snow off the driveway for as long as they can, it is a perfect way to burn calories and build muscle. Before you hit the snow, however, remember to stretch out your back and arms to prevent getting hurt.

1.   With your hands interlocked, reach for the sky and hold for ten minutes. Release and lock your fingers together behind your back, bringing your arms up without hurting yourself.

2.   Then stretch your triceps by bringing one arm over and behind your head and putting slight pressure on your elbow with the other hand. Switch sides.

3.   To stretch your back and hamstrings, release your upper body towards the floor, keeping legs as straight as possible and relaxing your back.

When you start shoveling, you can pick up the speed and do a great cardio workout. Remember however to keep your back firm, even when slightly bent over, and lift from a squat position which will work your legs and prevent straining your back. When you throw the snow, twist your upper body slightly, but in a controlled manner by keeping your abs firm and throwing the snow by concentrating on your arm muscles. Switch arms if you can, even if you feel like you have less control so you can work the muscles on both sides.

Workout #1: Sprint and Medicine Ball

Equipment: treadmill, medicine ball.

1.   Warm Up: Uphill treadmill walk for 3 minutes
Beginners: Incline 1.0
Intermediate: Incline 2.5
Advanced: Incline 4

2.   Sprint: Increase the treadmill speed to a sprint for 1 minute at 60%
Beginner: Incline 0
Intermediate: Incline .5
Advanced: Incline 1

3.   Recovery: Bring speed down to a walking pace for 30 seconds.

4.   Sprint: Increase the treadmill speed to a sprint for 1 minute at 80%, at incline 0.

5.   Recovery: Bring speed down to a walking pace for 30 seconds. Get off the treadmill.

6.   Squat Jump: Stand with back straight, legs apart, and squat pushing your glutes out. Jump up into the air and recuperate the squatting position.
Beginner: 10 reps
Intermediate: 15 reps
Advanced: 20 reps

7. Recovery: Shake your legs and catch your breath for 30 sec.

8.   Sprint: Get back on the treadmill and sprint for 2 minutes at 80%, at incline 0.

9.   Recovery: Bring speed down to a walking pace for 30 seconds. Get off the treadmill.

9.   Overhead Side Crunches: Hold a medicine ball straight overhead with your legs hip-width apart, and, looking straight ahead, shift your upper body over to one side, then the other side.
Beginner: 5 reps each side
Intermediate: 10 reps each side
Advanced: 20 reps each side

10.   Sprint: Get back on the treadmill and sprint for 3 minutes at 80%, at incline 0.

11.   Recovery: Bring speed down to a walking pace for 30 seconds. Get off the treadmill.

12.   Triceps Medicine Ball Extensions: Get off the treadmill and stand with legs hip-width apart, holding the medicine ball straight overhead. Keeping elbows in, lower the medicine ball behind your head.

Beginner: 10 reps
Intermediate: 15 reps
Advanced: 20 reps

Repeat the cycle 2, 3 times, resting 5 minutes in between each cycle for beginners, 1-2 minutes for intermediate, 1 minute for advanced.

Workout #2: Sprints and Weights

Equipment: 5-10lb dumbbells.

1.   Warm Up: Uphill treadmill walk for 3 minutes
Beginners: Incline 1.0
Intermediate: Incline 2.5
Advanced: Incline 4
2.   Sprint: Increase the treadmill speed to a sprint for 1 minute at 80%
Beginner: Incline 0
Intermediate: Incline .5
Advanced: Incline 1
3.   Recovery: Bring speed down to a walking pace for 30 seconds
4.   Sprint: Increase the treadmill speed to a sprint for 1 minute at 80%, at incline 0.
5.   Recovery: Bring speed down to 30% for 30 seconds. Get off the treadmill.
6.   Overhead Presses: Stand with your feet hip-width apart with two 5-10lb dumbbells in each hand. Bring arms up to your shoulders with your elbows bent at 90°. Bring the weights together overhead.
Beginner: Repeat 10 times.
Intermediate: Repeat 15 times.
Advanced: Repeat 20 times.
7.   Sprint: Increase the treadmill speed to a sprint for 1 minute at 80%, at incline 0.
8.   Recovery: Bring speed down to 30% for 30 seconds. Get off the treadmill.
9.   Pushups: Do one set of pushups:
Beginner: Repeat 10 times
Intermediate: Repeat 15 times
Advanced: Repeat 20 times
10.   Sprint: Get back on the treadmill and sprint for 3 minutes at 80%, at incline 0.
11.   Recovery: Bring speed down to a walking pace.

Repeat the cycle 2, 3 times, resting 5 minutes in between each cycle for beginners, 1-2 minutes for intermediate, 1 minute for advanced.

Workout #4: Full Treadmill HIIT

1.   Warm Up: Uphill treadmill walk for 3 minutes
Beginners: Incline 1.0
Intermediate: Incline 2.5
Advanced: Incline 4

2.   Sprint: Increase the treadmill speed to a sprint for 1 minute at 80%
Beginner: Incline 0
Intermediate: Incline .5
Advanced: Incline 1

3.   Recovery: Bring speed down to a 30% for 30 seconds

4.   Sprint: 2 minutes at 70%

5.   Recovery: 30% for 30 seconds

6.   Sprint: 2 minutes at 70% with 2 lb. dumbbells in each hand

7.   Recovery: 30% for 30 seconds

8.   Sprint: 3 minutes at 60%

9.   Recovery: 30 seconds at 20%

10.   Sprint: 3 minutes at 60% with dumbbells in each hand

11.   Recovery: 20 seconds at 20%

12. Cool down.

5 THE SIX SECRET WAYS TO ACHIEVING YOUR NEW YEAR'S RESOLUTIONS

For most people, New Year's resolutions are merely lies they tell themselves in order to feel good about the coming year. Don't be like them! Stop the cycle of excitement, failure, and disappointment. There are ways to make resolutions that stick, and we will teach you the six most effective.

Below are six approaches to setting resolutions you can actually feel excited about and are more likely to achieve.

Be Specific

"I want to lose weight" is vague and not very inspiring. What does it exactly mean to "lose weight"? Define a specific objective, such as: "I want to lose 4lbs a month, until June." Such a specific goal is will require you to focus on your diet and exercise regime and it isn't as daunting as "losing weight." It's measurable and you will be able to get excited about the outcome.

Another favorite resolution and equally as vague is "I want to get fit". Again, this is not specific enough to mean anything. Ask yourself, "What would it mean if I achieved [insert goal]?" and "What will the evidence be that I have achieved this goal?" Questions like these force you to focus on tangible outcomes rather than undefined wishes.

Focus on "Doing"

A useful way to be more specific is to convert every "being" goal into a measurable "doing" goal. Generally there are three types of goals: Being, Doing and Having. Doing goals are self-explanatory — "I want to surf the big waves in Hawaii" is an example. Being goals are more nebulous.

"I want to be fit" isn't really a goal.

"Run a 5k in under an hour" is a goal you can really get behind.

Remember that "being" is really an outcome of "doing". Being fit is the result of working out and eating good quality food.

Small, Early Wins

Make sure that you set some small steps that you can cross off the list at the start of your goal pursuit. Early wins are highly motivating. Casinos use this principle every day to make sure people keep spending money. If you have an early win on a slot machine you're more likely to stick around and spend more money.

Create momentum early on by stacking daily and weekly "wins" one after the other and you'll feel the exhilaration to keep going.

Record Everything

"Quantified self" is the buzz term thrown around these days for what is really just tracking progress towards goals. Recording your daily efforts is a great way to ensure you are always able to make measurable progress towards your goals. Gathering objective data can help you realize what is working and what might need to change.

Above all though, it is fantastic to be able to see your progress right in front of you. Nothing is more motivating than seeing tangible evidence of your success.

There are several mobile phone apps out there to help you track your progress towards goals. Perhaps one of the better apps out there for Android and Apple devices is Lift. The app allows you to input your goals, timelines and helps you plan the necessary daily activities. Like Lift, various apps offer features to track your goals and chart your progress. It's up to you to stay dedicated to using them!

Raise the Stakes

It is one thing to make a silent resolution to yourself, but if you're really committed, tell someone else about it. Research shows conclusively that we are more likely to achieve what we set out to do by making our intentions public. You don't need to tell the whole world (although social media can often be useful). Tell someone close to you who will keep you honest and on track. Now, you're accountable for making it happen and you'll feel a lot more internal motivation to achieve it.

Finally — Don't Try to Do Too Much

Focus is a powerful thing. People who want to achieve goals but repeatedly fail to make progress are often trying to do too much. Your time, attention, energy and interest can only go so far. By pursuing only two or three goals at any one time you make sure your effort is focused like a laser beam!

For instance, you might want to be able to deadlift 350lbs, learn basic Spanish, make some extra money, learn guitar and build a shed in your backyard. Some of these are doable alongside other goals but trying to do all of them at once is a recipe for failure. Instead, prioritize, and figure out what you most want to accomplish first.

Sometimes simplifying and planning to achieve small things is better than over-reaching. People who are generally regarded as successful have a single-minded focus about achieving one thing. Just remember that whatever you want should

31

contribute to the well-being of your life and shouldn't negatively impact yourself and those around you.

Make productive use of your time and be sure to take responsibility for your life and you can't go wrong. Let's make this year really count!.

6 FEBRUARY

February has come around and the coldest of the winter has passed. You don't want yet another year to go by without following through with your fitness resolutions so it is important to stay consistent with your HIIT routines. HIIT workouts are great to keep warm, get the heart pumping and building lean muscle.

Also, don't forget Valentine's Day is coming up and whether you want to look and feel good for that special someone, or simply for yourself, find the motivation to pick up the intensity in each exercise.

This month, we will be encouraging you to pick up some winter sports, as well as walking you through your daily workout with free weights, an indoor rowing machine, resistance band, Swiss ball and a jump rope. There is a bonus couple workout you can do with your special someone as well!

Tip of the Month: Winter Sports

Just because it is snowing and cold doesn't mean you have to stay indoors. Sports like snow skiing, snowboarding, and hockey were made for the cold. Even if you don't have any experience, there are plenty of beginner classes that are fun to take up with friends. You would be surprised at how fun it is, and how sore you feel the next day! Whatever sport you choose, keep in mind that you need to dress right for the occasion, keep hydrated, even though it is cold, and warm up and cool down to prevent straining your muscles.

Workout #1: Indoor Rowing

The rowing machine is a great calorie buster. It may not be a good exercise though if you have:

- symptomatic low back pain, or a history of symptomatic intervertebral disc pathology;

- hip pain of any sort;

- an aberrant posture;

- of if you sit all day.

How to row:
- For your first row, set the resistance to "low" while you figure out your form, then slowly ramp it up on subsequent rows.

- Secure your feet on the pads with the straps tight enough so your feet don't move around as you slide.

- Bring your knees up and slide to the top of the machine. Grab the handle using an overhand grip, but don't hold too tightly.

- Pull the handle with you as you slide to the end of the machine. Your legs should be straight, but knees should still have a slight bend in them so they aren't locked.

- Lean back slightly and pull your hands up to your chest, holding the handle so it is right below your breasts, with elbows pointing down against your sides. This is the position where you should begin your workout, and it's also your ending position once you complete a full stroke

1.   Warm up: Row at a comfortable pace for 1-2 minutes.
2.   At the end of the second minute explode into maximum effort in 60 seconds.
3.   Slow down for 30 sec.
4.   Speed up at max effort for 60 seconds.
5.   Slow down for 30 sec.
6.   Speed up at max effort for 60 seconds.
7.   Slow down for 30 sec
8. Speed up at max effort for 60 seconds.
9. Slow down for 30 sec
10. Speed up at max effort for 60 seconds.
11. Cool down for 5 min. Row at a comfortable pace

If you are a beginner you can rest up to 60 sec. If you are advanced take shorter rests 15-30 sec.

Workout #2: Jump Rope and Free Weights

Equipment: jump rope, dumbbells or any other weight. If you are home you can use bottles filled with water, for example.

Tip: You may want to try a cordless jump rope for this workout, since it will give you the same great focus on cardio while not distracting you as it hits your feet.

1.   Warm up: trotting with your jump rope, warm up at 20% for 2 minutes
2.   Jump Rope: Pick up to a 90% intensity for 1 minute
3.   Recovery: Bring it back down to 20% for 1 minute
4.   Biceps Flex: Put your jump rope aside and hold a weight in each hand. Bend your knees into a slight squat with your weights right above your thighs and alternate lifting each weight up to your shoulder, without losing your squat position.
Beginner: 10 reps
Intermediate: 15 reps
Advanced: 20 reps
5.   Jump Rope: for 1 minute at 90%
6.   Recovery: for 1 minute at 20%
7.   Squat and Shoulder Lift: Stand with your feet a little wider than hip-width apart and hold a weight in each hand resting at your side. Squat as low as you can without lifting your heels or losing your balance, keeping your back straight, shifted forward. At the same time lift your arms straight out until they reach shoulder height. As you straighten your legs bring down the weights and repeat.
Beginner: 10 reps
Intermediate: 15 reps
Advanced: 20 reps

Repeat the cycle without warm up 2, 3 times, resting 5 minutes in between each cycle for beginners, 1-2 minutes for intermediate, 1 minute for advanced.

Workout #3: Indoor Rowing Based on Distance

1. Warm up: Row 100m at a 20% intensity
2. 100m: Row 100m at an 80% intensity
3. 50m: Row at a 30% intensity
4. 200m: Row at an 70% intensity
5. 50m: Row at a 30% intensity
6. 300m: Row at a 70% intensity
7. 50m: Row at a 20% intensity
8. 200m: Row at a 60% intensity
9. 50m: Row at a 20% intensity
10. 100m: Row at a 90% intensity
- .100m: Row at a 30% intensity
11. Cool down.

Workout #4: Valentine's Day Couple Workout

Even if you don't have a significant other, you can do this with your friends! It is just as fun and effective, and maybe even more so!

Equipment: jump rope, Swiss ball.

1. Warm up: trotting with your jump rope, warm up at 20% for 2 minutes
2. Jump Rope: Pick up to a 90% intensity for 1 minute
3. Recovery: Bring it back down to 20% for 1 minute
4. Swiss Ball Crunch and Overhead Toss: as you do crunches on a Swiss ball, hold a medicine ball overhead, tossing it to your partner as you come up. You partner should toss it back to you as you go back down onto the Swiss ball and repeat.
Beginners: 15 reps
Intermediate: 25 reps
Advanced: 35 reps
5. Squat Jump: Synchronization is key with this couples squat jump. With each of you holding one end of a resistance band, stand far enough apart for the band to pull slightly. At the same time, jump as high as you can, and lower back into squat position as you land.
Beginners: 10 reps
Intermediate: 20 reps
Advanced: 30 reps
6. Partner Jump and Drops: One partner lies on the floor. The other partner jumps over the midsection of his or her partner, turns around and jumps back. He or she quickly lies down on the floor as the other partner gets up to take his/her turn at jumping.
7. Cool down: jumping rope at 30% for 3 minutes.

Rest for 1-5 minutes and repeat the cycle 3-4 times.

Top.me

7 WHAT'S THE MOST EFFICIENT CARDIO WORKOUT?

There are times when you just don't feel like doing a HIIT workout. But what other cardio exercise gets you the most bang for the buck?

Running

Running is a full body workout and the amount of calories it burns per hour varies dramatically from person to person, depending on how fast you run, on what surface and your technique/stride. Generally, you can expect to burn 600-1200 calories per hour.

Even walking on a treadmill can burn up to 400 calories an hour, although the more breathless you feel and the more aerobic the treadmill workout, the more calories you'll get rid of! If you run on a treadmill, try setting an incline (hill run), which boosts your metabolism and add interval training (i.e. walk, jog and sprint at various times to mix it up). Sprinting, even for bursts of 20-30 seconds, dramatically boosts your metabolism rate.

Cycling

The motion of pedaling uses the powerful muscles in your

leg and burns calories quickly. The number of calories you burn will depend on the intensity in which you cycle, but generally cycling can burn 500-1000 calories per hour and is one of the highest calories burners out there, especially if done correctly.

Don't forget that cycling outside adds the elements of the wind resistance etc and adds to an even more intense workout, but if you don't fancy facing the changeable weather, a stationary bike can be just as effective. If you choose to use the bike at a gym, make sure you set the resistance high enough, so that you use the power in your legs, as opposed to the natural pedaling motion, it might feel easy, but it is cheating! If you are breathing rapidly, it is a good indication that you have the settings just right!

The bonus of stationary bikes, is the fact that you can keep a check of the distance you have cycled over and for how long, allowing you to track your workout and calorie loss. A tip for cycling is to do 2-3 minutes of intense pedaling and then rest (pedal slower for a few minutes). This high intensity workout will ensure that you keep losing calories after your workout, rather than if you exercise at a slower, steady pace throughout. Joining a spinning class is a good way to get some high-intensity workouts in to music and a nice sociable environment, with instructions from a trained professional.

Elliptical Trainer

Contrary to popular belief, the elliptical trainer is not the most effective gym machine for burning calories, especially if you tend to hold the handrail for support when working out. You can expect to burn approximately 600 calories per hour and more if the trainer includes arm movements.

The reason you burn less than running is that the machine does a lot of the work for you with its momentum, rather than your muscles having to do the majority of the power/movement. To get the most from your workout on this machine, put the resistance at a higher setting and don't use the rails to lean on for support, this way you will burn more calories and build up your endurance.

Rowing Machine

The rowing machine is hard work for the body, and most exercise that feels tough is usually excellent for calories burning and fitness goals! The good news is, that this all-over body worker burns over 1000 calories per hour. The rower works your upper and lower body and is not only great for warming up, but for a longer, more intense workout.

The motion can get a little monotonous, so a good way to keep at it and keep burning through those calories is to change the speeds at different intervals. It is important to use the correct technique when rowing, to avoid back and knee injury, so if in doubt, ask your gym instructor. As well as limiting injury, using the right technique will ensure that your body is working in its optimum condition for calories busting.

Stair Climber

If you add resistance to the stair climber, you can burn approximately 600 calories in an hour and work on your lower-body strength. The muscles it uses are limited, so adding some dumbbell lifting can add to the effectiveness of the workout.

Jump Rope/Skipping

There's a reason Rocky trains with a skipping rope! This is one of the simplest and most effective workouts you can do to use your whole body, improve your cardiovascular endurance and your strength, speed and agility. It can burn over 750 calories an hour, although an hour of jumping can be pretty intense, but even adding 10 minutes to your gym session will reap rewards.

Kettlebell Workout

Researchers at the University of Wisconsin published a

study[11] that proved that a 20 minutes kettlebell workout burn around 270 cal. Volunteers performed a pre-determined 20-minute kettlebell snatch workout typical of a common kettlebell routine. The workout consisted of a brief warm-up, then 15 seconds of snatches, followed by 15 seconds of rest. The study found that they were burning approximately 20.2 calories per minute! So grab your kettlebell and go for a snatch to do your cardio in half the time!

Which is the Best Cardio Workout for You?

At the end of the day, the cardio you enjoy the most, will mean you are more likely to stick at it and do it consistently every day. The best option is to choose some exercises that you both enjoy and benefit from, and mix them up in your gym routine to keep it fresh. Your body will respond better if you switch things around, mix the exercises up and add some obstacles, such as weight (dumbbells) or higher resistance.

Exercise classes, with an instructor, friends and some music blasting, are great ways to burn calories – often without really feeling like you're suffering too much! Try a step aerobics class and burn around 800 calories in an hour, as well as tone specific areas of your body.

Team sports such as basketball and football are great forms of exercise, as is martial arts. A racquet sport with a friend can be a great social activity and an intense workout, with the quick movements and changes of pace, as well as competitive edge all helping lose some weight. If you want to try something a bit different, rock climbing can burn up to 800 calories an hour and uses a lot of arm and leg strength and bursts of power.

---

[11] http://www.acefitness.org/acefit/expert-insight-article/47/2982/kettlebells-twice-the-results-in-half-the/

New Year, New You

8 MARCH

It is still cold outside, and in some places you might even be getting some fresh snow. Luckily this month is also St. Patrick's Day, so we have a fun tip and some great indoor HIIT workouts for you to rotate.

The trainings can be intense in the moment, but as you build up resistance, you build strength and improve your cardiovascular capacity.

The March workouts are designed for a stationary bike. Rotate the four different workouts to build muscle as well as resistance.

Tip of the Month: Shamrock Protein Shake

This month, hold the Shamrock Shakes if you don't want to gain back some of those freshly-lost holiday pounds. Instead, make up your own Shamrock Protein Shake to support your workouts and curb your sugar cravings. Here is the recipe:

½ cup low-fat cottage cheese
¼ cup protein powder (you can use vanilla or plain)
¼ tsp. mint extract
4-5 mint leaves

2-3 packs pure stevia
4 oz. water
¼ frozen banana
1 tbs. sugar-free instant pistachio pudding mix
3 drops green food coloring

Mix all of the ingredients in a blender and enjoy!

Workout #1: HIIT on a Stationary Bike with Strength Building:

(Designed for standard bikes with a 1- 20 resistance level)

1. Warm up: 2 minutes on 3
3. 1 minute on 8
4. 1 minute on 10
5. 1 minute on 12

6. 1 minute on 4
7. 1 minute on 7
8. 1 minute on 9
9. 1 minute on 11
10. 1 minute on 13

11. 1 minute on 4
12. 1 minute on 8
13. 1 minute on 10
14. 1 minute on 12
15. 1 minute on 14

16. 1 minute on 4
17. 1 minute on 11
18. 1 minute on 13
19. 1 minute on 15
20. Cool down: 3 minutes on 3

For beginners, if it's hard to bike go a step down for each interval, and for advanced, go up 1-2 levels at each level except for the warm up and cool down.

Workout #2: Flat Belly HIIT

1. Warm up: Stationary bike at level 4 for 3 minutes
2. Stationary Bike: 2 minute at level 8
3. Ski Twists: Get off the stationary bike and do 50 Ski Twists. Beginners can do 20.

You're jumping as you would with jumping jacks, but this time you're keeping your feet together and twisting at the hips rather than throwing the arms. Simply jump and twist to the left, then back to the center, then twist right and back to the center.

4. Bicycle Crunches: do 50 of them. Beginners can do 20.
5. Stationary Bike: 2 minutes at level 8
6. Get off the stationary bike and do Vertical Hip Lifts for 60 sec.
7. Side Plank 60 sec each side (advanced), 30 sec each side (beginners)
8. Plank Jumping Jacks. Jump and separate your legs until they form a Y with your body. Jump your feet together. Continue for 30 sec (beginners), 60 sec (advanced)
9. Mountain Climbers. 30 sec (beginners), 60 sec (advanced)
10. Stationary Bike: 2 minutes at level 8
11. Side Plank 30-60 sec each side
12. Plank Jumping Jacks 30-60 sec.
13. Cool down: Stationary bike at level 4 for 3 minutes

Rest for 5 minutes and repeat cycle 3-4 times.

Workout #3: Intermittent Stationary Bike Workout

1. Warm up: 2 minutes at level 1
2. 2 minutes at level 2
3. 2 minutes at level 3
4. 1 minute at level 8
5. 1 minute at level 4
6. 2 minutes at level 8
7. 2 minutes at level 4
8. 2 minutes at level 9
9. 2 minutes at level 5
10. 2 minutes at level 10
11. 2 minutes at level 6
12. 2 minutes at level 3
13. Cool down: 1 minute at level 1

Beginners, for the high levels, start one level down, and for advanced spinners, start one level up. Rest for 5 minutes and repeat cycle 3 times.

Workout #4: Hyper Intense HIIT Stationary Bike Workout

Resistance: 3 for beginners, 4-5 for intermediate, and 6-7 for advanced. Speeds should be around 75-90 RPM for the HIIT, and down 45-60 for the recovery.

1. 15 seconds HIIT – 15 seconds recovery
2. 15 seconds HIIT – 15 seconds recovery
3. 30 seconds HIIT – 30 seconds recovery
4. 45 seconds HIIT – 45 seconds recovery
5. 60 seconds HIIT – 60 seconds recovery
6. 60 seconds HIIT – 60 seconds recovery
7. 60 seconds HIIT – 60 seconds recovery
8. 45 seconds HIIT – 45 seconds recovery
9. 45 seconds HIIT – 45 seconds recovery
10. 30 seconds HIIT – 30 seconds recovery
11. 30 seconds HIIT – 30 seconds recovery
12. 15 seconds HIIT – 15 seconds recovery
13. 15 seconds HIIT – 15 seconds recovery

9 SEVEN WAYS TO BEAT YOUR CRAVINGS

No matter how diligent you are with your diet, you may still find yourself craving for unhealthy foods. Before you give in to temptation, here are six questions to ask yourself.

Are You Craving the Food for Emotional Reasons?

Often you crave certain foods when you are in some sort of emotional distress, and often the type of food you crave is related to the emotion you are experiencing. For example, often one craves salty, crunchy snacks (e.g. potato crisps or pretzels) when one is frustrated, irritated or angry. Similarly one may crave for rich, creamy, soft, starchy snacks (e.g. cake or ice cream) when one is depressed or lonely.

What you need to remember in this situation is that the food will not compensate the emotional pain you are feeling. Deal with your emotions at hand rather than turning to food as a means to block out or avoid the issue.

Are You Actually Thirsty?

People mistake thirst for hunger. Try drinking a glass of water, wait ten minutes and see if the craving has subsided.

Are You Eating Correctly?

Cravings can be our body's way of telling us what we need. In order to prevent cravings, you need to make sure that you are getting a healthy, balanced diet with a variety of foods from the five different food groups – dairy products (e.g. milk, yogurt), meat and meat alternatives (e.g. chicken, fish, beef, eggs, legumes), fruits and vegetables, fats and oils (e.g. margarine, sunflower oil, avocados, nuts and seeds) and the breads, cereals and grains group (e.g. bread, rice, pasta, breakfast cereals, potatoes).

Are You Exercising Enough?

Exercise can help to prevent and manage cravings. So, if you find yourself with a craving that you just can't ignore, go to the gym, or go for a run. You may find that after few minutes of doing something positive for your body, the craving has disappeared.

Can You Distract Yourself?

Sometimes you crave food because you are bored. Maybe you just need to be occupy your mind with something else. Try writing down alternatives to eating. This list could include exercising (see above), phoning a friend, taking a bubble bath, reading a book or a magazine, or even tidying up a particularly messy closet.

Can You Substitute the Craved Food for Another?

Often you can satisfy a craved food with a healthier alternative. For example, gherkins instead of crisps, or low fat frozen yoghurt instead of ice cream.

If Nothing Else Will Do…

Sometimes, however, it is best to just have a little bit of what you are craving rather than avoiding eating it completely and then eventually going on a binge. Often, the first bite and the last bite of a food are the only ones we pay attention to.

Have only a small portion – just enough to satisfy your craving. Focus on the food while you eat it and enjoy it. Don't let yourself feel guilty, discouraged, weak, or frustrated, because of it. After all we're all humans, and a little treat now and then does not hurt.

Top.me

10 NINE HIGHLY EFFECTIVE BODYWEIGHT EXERCISES TO TIGHTEN YOUR CORE, ARMS AND BUTT

You don't need a gym, fancy equipment, or heavy weights to get a toned body. With these 9 body weight exercises, you'll be rocking your core, arms and butt.

Let's get to work! Do two rounds of this routine. In each set, beginners perform 5-8 reps, and advanced athletes perform 10-15 reps. Or simply fit any of the exercises into your regular workout.

Single Leg Deadlift

Main Muscle: Hamstrings, glutes, abdominal

Directions:

- Stand on one leg.
- Perform a stiff legged deadlift by bending at the hip, extending your free leg behind you for balance.
- Continue lowering your arms until you are

parallel to the ground, and then return to the upright position bringing your leg and arms together.

- Repeat with the other leg.

Pike Push-Up

Main Muscle: Shoulders

Directions:

- Start from a classic pushup position.
- Keep your legs straight and walk your hands back so you are in a pike position.
- Your upper body and lower body should be at about a 90 degree angle.
- Extend the arms overhead so that they are in line with your spine and reaching straight out from the shoulders. That part is important because it is that position that works the shoulders.
- Contract the core.
- Bend the elbows and lower yourself down until your head almost contacts the ground.
- Press back up.

Hyperextension

Main Muscle: Back

Directions:

- Lie face down on the platform (a hyperextension bench, or Swiss Ball) tucking your ankles securely under the footpads.
- Adjust so your upper thighs lie flat leaving enough room for you to bend at the waist without any restriction.
- With your body straight, keep your arms up on the

sides (can be in front of you bent or behind your head). This will be your starting position.

- Start bending forward slowly at the waist as far as you can while keeping your back flat bringing your arms forward. Inhale as you perform this movement. Keep moving forward until you feel a nice stretch on the hamstrings and you can no longer keep going without a rounding of the back.

Tip: Never round the back as you perform this exercise. Also, some people can go farther than others. The key thing is that you go as far as your body allows you to without rounding the back.

- Slowly raise your torso back to the initial position as you inhale. Tip: Avoid the temptation to arch your back past a straight line. Also, do not swing the torso at any time in order to protect the back from injury.

Repeat for the recommended amount of repetitions.

One Arm Push-Up

Maine Muscle: Chest

Directions:

- Begin lying prone on the ground. Move yourself into a position supporting your weight on your toes and one arm. Your working arm should be placed directly under the shoulder, fully extended. Your legs should be extended, and for this movement you may need a wider base, placing your feet further apart than in a normal push-up.
- Maintain good posture, and place your free hand behind your back. This will be your starting position.
- Lower yourself by allowing the elbow to flex until

you touch the ground.

- Descend slowly, and reverse direction be extending the arm to return to the starting position.

Single Leg Dip

Main Muscle: Triceps

Directions:

- Sit on the edge of a bench or chair or any other stable platform with your arms at your sides and feet flat on the ground.
- Grip the edge of the bench. Keep your arms close to the body.
- Slowly slide your body off the bench so you are suspended by your arms behind you. You may need to walk your feet away from the bench a few inches for comfort.
- Elevate one leg and extend it straight in front of you.
- Bend your arms and slowly lower your body toward the ground until your arms are bent to 90 degrees. Make sure your arms are straight behind you and do not let them flare out to the sides.
- Push down with your arms to lift your body to the starting position. Do not completely lock your elbows; keep them slightly bent as you reach the top of the motion.

Complete the set and switch legs.

Pike Elbow Up

Main Muscle: Shoulders

Directions:

- Start from a classic pushup position.
- Keep your legs straight and walk your hands back so you are in a pike position.
- Your upper body and lower body should be at about a 90 degree angle.
- Extend the arms overhead so that they are in line with your spine and reaching straight out from the shoulders. That part is important because it is that position that works the shoulders.
- Contract the core.
- Bend the elbows and lower yourself down until they contacts the ground.
- Press back up.

Explosive Long Jump

Main Muscle: Legs

Directions:

- Start in the upright position.
- Bend your knees in a jumping position.
- Push yourself explosively forward.

Triceps Extension Push-Up

Main Muscle: Triceps

Directions:

- Begin lying prone on the ground. Move yourself into a position supporting your weight on your toes and arms.
- Set your hands further than your head.
- Lower yourself down, bending only at the elbows.
- Extend back up.

Single Leg Hip Thrust

Main Muscle: Glutes

Directions:

- Lie on the floor with your arms along your body.
- Raise your off-leg up and straighten it in line with your other thigh.
- Pressing through your heel and firing your glutes, lift your hips off the floor. Your weight should rest on your heel and your upper back – not your toes or your neck and cervical spine. Extend your hips until they form a straight line with your knees and shoulders.
- Make sure the end range of motion comes from the hips – squeezing the glutes together at the top of the movement – and not from hyperextension.
- Change the leg.

11 APRIL

The weather really wants to start getting warmer, and you might even get some days where you get to leave your snow boots at home! With the rain, however, you might have to take out those rain boots and keep your all-weather jacket on.

This month, we keep up the HIIT rhythm and take one of the workouts outdoors. After many months of working out indoors, some fresh air and cool breeze might do you good, at the very least to get a peek at the spring flowers and melting snow. We will also give you some tips on how to make the most out of your spring cleaning and burn some extra calories as you sift through things to keep and give away.

Tip of the Month: Spring Cleaning

It's that time of the year again! The spring cleaning annual ritual is not only the perfect time to clean the deepest and darkest corners of your house and get rid of unwanted things that take up space, it can also be a time for renewal. Here are some tips you can consider to make Spring Cleaning part of your daily workout:

- Get in some old workout clothes as you clean to get you in the mood.
- Put on some music and shake it!

- Stay hydrated – when cleaning up you tend to lose fluids but because you don't think you are exercising, you often forget to drink enough water
- Don't be afraid to put away the Swiffer and get on your hands and knees. There are plenty of gadgets that have made all of our lives easier when it comes to keeping our house clean. But when the goal is to get in a work out, don't be shy about bringing out the scrub brush.
- Baskets of things (clothes, shoes, books, spices) make great weights. Do a couple a squats before taking it to Good Will.

Workout #1:

1.   High Knees: Run in place bringing your knees as high as you can at a warm-up pace for 20 seconds
2.   High Knees: Pump up the speed to as fast as you can for 20 seconds
3.   Squats: With your legs hip-width apart, lower into a squat while bringing your arms straight out in front of you.
Beginner: 15 times
Intermediate: 25 times
Advanced 30 times
4.   Burpees: Start standing with your legs hip-width apart and crouch down with your hands on the floor in front of you. Jump your legs back until you are in a pushup position and quickly jump your legs back under your body. Stand up again with your arms at your side. Do 20 as fast as you can
Rest for 1 minute.

For beginners: repeat 5 times, resting in between each round.
For intermediates: 10 rounds.
And for advanced: 15 rounds. Rest less between rounds.

Workout #2: Outside sprints

Note: This workout can be performed outside or inside where there is space to sprint 50m.

1. Warm up: Jog for 2 minutes at a 20% intensity
2. Sprint: 30 seconds at a 90% intensity
3. Jog: 30-60 sec at 20%
4. High Knees: 20 seconds at 90%
5. Jog: 30-60 sec at 20%
6. Sprint for 30 seconds at 90%
7. Jumping Jacks: 30-60 sec
8. Jog: for 1 minute at 20%
7. Sprint for 30 seconds at 90%
8. Squats: 30-60 sec

Rest for 2 minutes and repeat:
Beginners: 5 rounds
Intermediates: 8 rounds.
Advanced: 10 rounds.
Rest in between each round.

Workout #3: Stationary HIIT

1. Warm up: Jumping Jacks for 2 minutes
2. Squats: 20 squats
3. Side leg raises: standing with feet hip-width apart, lift your right leg to your side as high as you can, without bending your knees. Do 20 on one side, then 20 on the other side.
4. Toe tap jumps: standing with feet hip-width apart, bring one leg up to the opposite hand, and switch legs as fast as you can. Continue for 1 minute
5. Lunge Kicks: From full lunge position, push yourself up with your back leg and use the momentum from that same leg to kick up as high as you can. Lower back down into lunge position. Do 20 on each side.
6. Jumping jacks: as fast as you can without losing form for 1 minute. Then lower the speed to 30 seconds.
7. Climbers: Start in plank position, but with your hips slightly raised. Bring up one of your legs up to your chest and back down again, switching your legs immediately. Do 30 times

Rest for 2 minutes and repeat:
Beginner 3 times
Intermediate 5 times
Advanced 7-8 times.

Top.me

12 MAY

You've made it through the winter! Flowers are starting to pop out of the ground and leaves grow on the trees. In light of nature's renewal, it is a perfect time for renewing your commitment to your fitness and health through practicing at least one of these routines every day of the month.

This month we have some exercises that will work your core and take you outside to the track to get your cardio in.

Tip of the Month: Gardening and Yard Work

This might seem strange to you, but gardening is a surprisingly good workout! You could burn up to 600 calories per hour doing gardening and landscaping in your own yard. Heavy yard work is the best, and includes landscaping, moving rocks, and hauling dirt. Gardening, including planting flowers and pulling weeds can burn up to 400 calories per hour, and mowing the lawn can burn up to 350 calories per hour. Don't shy away from getting down and dirty preparing your yard for spring and summer.

If you are new to gardening, try some vegetables that are relatively easy to grow like tomatoes, zucchini or peppers. If you prefer flowers instead, you can try planting some annuals like marigolds, impatiens or sunflowers, or some perennials like pansies, daylilies and sage. When you buy your seeds or plants, ask the specialist about special care, how often you should water your plant, what kind of fertilizer you need, and whether it should be in direct sunlight. You'll feel very proud of yourself and feel fitter when your masterpiece is finished!

Workout #1: HIIT on the Track

1. Warm up: Two laps or 2 min around the track.
2. 20 high-knee marching steps
3. 20 butt-kickers
4. 60 sec sprint
5. Skip for 1 lap or 30 sec
6. 20 heel walks
7. 20 toe walks
8. 60 sec sprint
9. Skip for 1 lap or 30 sec

Repeat 1-3 times, depending on conditioning level. Stretch when you are done.

Workout #2: HIIT Sprinting

1. Jog 1 lap or 2 min
2. Sprint 30 sec
3. Recover 15-30 sec
4. Sprint 30 sec
5. Recover v
6. Sprint 30 sec
7. Recover 15-30 sec

Rest for 2-3 minutes and repeat:
Beginner: 1 round
Intermediate: 2 rounds
Advanced: 3 rounds
Remember to stretch when you are done.

Workout #3: Inside/Outside Quick Intervals

1. Jog in place or jog around a track for 30 seconds
2. Mountain Climbers: In a pushup position, bend your right leg and move it up on the ground towards your chest while moving your left hand up at the same time. Move your body forward. Alternate hand and feet so your are moving forward as fast as you can for 20 seconds
3. Jog in place or around a track for 30 seconds
4. Squats: With your legs hip-width apart, squat down to the ground keeping your back straight, at the same time bringing your arms straight up to shoulder height. As you straighten your legs again, bring your hands down by your side. Repeat for 20 seconds.
5. Jog in place or around the track for 30 seconds.
6. Jump Squats: With your feet together and arms elbows bent, close to your body, jump your feet out to the side (a little wider than hip-width apart) and squat down. Come back up and jump feet back together. Continue for 20 seconds
7. Jog in place or around the track for 30 seconds
8. Walking Lunges: Standing feet together with your hands on your hips lunge with one leg forward so when you go down your forward leg is in a 90-degree angle with your foot. Push yourself up with the other leg and step forward. Continue for 20 seconds.
9. Jog in place or around the track for 1 minute.

Repeat once if you are a beginner, twice if you are at an intermediate level, and three times if you are advanced.

Top.me

13 FIVE HEALTHY SUMMER TIME COOK OUT IDEAS

Now that we are approaching the summer months, it is time to fire up the grill and have some great cook outs! Cook outs can be such a fun time with family, friends and loved ones! Since the summer time is also representative of beach season, it is important that we are eating the right foods when we cook out.

Fortunately for you, the grill is one of the best ways to eat healthy and also add in some bold flavors! When you are cooking out, you should make sure to stay away from the fatty protein sources such as hot dogs, hamburgers, and ribs. You are about to find out that there are delicious alternatives to these cook out meats.

These 5 healthy summer time cook out ideas will fill you up and may even help you lose weight. They will also satisfy your savory and sweet tooth in unique and delicious ways.

The next time that you cook out make sure to follow one of these cook out guides for a delicious and memorable experience!

Cook Out Idea 1: BBQ Grilled Chicken Breasts

Grilled Chicken Breasts Marinated with Bbq Sauce, Olive Oil, and Garlic
Grilled Pineapple with Fresh Honey Brushed on It
Grilled Green Beans, Broccoli and Cauliflower with Olive Oil and Fresh Pepper

This is a delicious and healthy meal that will fill you up with tons of the best source of lean protein and nutrients. Make sure that you buy the boneless skinless chicken breasts. The good thing about grilling is that sugar based sauces like BBQ marinade are mostly stripped of the sugar once they are off the grill, but you still get the flavor. BBQ makes for a great marinade because it has a smoky and sweet combination. Grilled pineapple brushed with honey makes for a sweet treat that you can enjoy guilt free. To grill veggies, simple wrap them in tin foil and brush some olive oil and seasoning on them!

Chicken breast BBQ marinade recipe:
This is healthy! We mix vinegar with some good quality olive oil. For about one cup of marinade (for 5-6 chicken breasts), we need:

3/4 cup olive oil (use a high quality one)
2 tablespoons balsamic vinegar
2 teaspoon salt
2 teaspoon white sugar
some dried oregano, basil, onion and garlic powder, some black or red pepper as to your liking

Mix all ingredients well together. That's it! Now just pour the BBQ marinade into a bag and add the chicken breasts. Let them rest for a few hours.

Cook Out Idea 2: Grilled Salmon

Grilled Salmon Marinated with Olive Oil, Lemon, and Dill
Grilled Asparagus Spears Marinated with Balsamic Vinegaratte, Olive Oil and Cracked Pepper
Grilled Sweet Potato Fries with Cinnamon

This is a great meal that combines a healthy source of protein and omega 3 fatty acids with the grilled salmon. Brush some olive oil, lemon and dill and the salmon is delicious on the grill! Grilled asparagus spears make for a healthy and delicious summertime treat and it's one of the best vegetarian protein sources. The combination of balsamic, olive oil and cracked pepper compliment this vegetable perfectly. To make the grilled sweet potato fries slice a sweet potato to your liking and sprinkle fresh cinnamon on it. Throw on the grill for about 30 minutes and you have a healthy alternative to regular fries.

Cook Out Idea 3: Grilled Sirloin Steak

Grilled Sirloin Steak
Grilled Baked Potato Spears
Grilled Cauliflower and Broccoli with Garlic and Honey

This is a high protein and carbohydrate meal that can really accelerate lean muscle gains without a lot of excess calories. And we are all as well aware of the importance of complex carbohydrates. Grilled Sirloin steak is one of the leanest cuts of steak and can be enjoyed guilt free in moderation. Sirloin steak is much leaner than filet mignon and other popular beef cuts. Grilled Cauliflower and Brocolli with garlic and honey is a fantastic complement to the sirloin steak. The combination of the garlic and honey makes these veggies a sweet and delicious summertime vegetable treat. Throw the veggies in some tin foil and throw on the grill for 15-20 minutes and these delicious veggies are ready for your next cook out.

Cook Out Idea 4: Grilled Pork Chops

Grilled Pork Chops

Grilled Pork Chops with Guava BBQ Sauce
Grilled Vidalia Onion Blossom
Grilled Sweet Potatoes with Cinnamon Butter and Marshmallow

Grilled pork chops are absolutely delicious on the grill. I recommend brushing on some guava BBQ sauce for a unique and protein packed summertime meal. This one will win over all of your friends and family. Vidalia onions are absolutely delicious on the grill. Simply season them as you like and peel the skin and they will be piping hot and delicious within 15 minutes. A much healthier alternative to the deep fried onions you will find at restaurants. The sweet potatoes are so delicious they can be eaten in place of dessert. Marshmallow and cinnamon butter complement the sweet potatoes for a deliciously and sweet combination.

Cook Out Idea 5: Grilled Turkey Burgers

Grilled Turkey Burgers on Whole Wheat Toasted Buns
Grilled Veggie Medley for Turkey Burger Fixings: Onions, Avocado, Tomatoes

This one is a personal favorite. Grilled turkey burgers on a whole wheat bun are a great alternative to the usual hot dogs and hamburgers that are enjoyed during cookouts in the summer. You will be saving over 300 calories per burger by swapping out the lean turkey burgers in place of the fatty beef that is typically used for cook outs. Grilled veggies such as onion, avocado, and tomatoes make these burgers colorful, unique and delicious. Avocado is one of the healthiest things you can consume, and gives you a big serving of healthy fats. Forget the cheese and condiments and decorate your burger with fresh veggies for a real summer time treat!

14 JUNE

The weather is starting to warm up and the layers are starting to coming off, so you want to look and feel your best!

How can High Intensity Interval Training help you do that? HIIT works by helping you balance the time between maximum intensity and rest and short intervals, making the most of your workout in a short amount of time.

How do you know when you are at maximum intensity? Find out what your target heart rate is and manage it through a heart rate device or by counting your heart beats during a rest or a low-intensity move. To really take advantage of our workouts, you want to hit about 85% of your maximum heart rate during high-intensity moves. However it is always important to check with your physician before carrying out any sort of physical activity.

This month, we will do a mix of indoor and outdoor workouts focused around jogging and plyometric strength building without the additional free weights.

Tip of the Month: Take Latin Dance Classes

Pick up some salsa, merengue, or samba classes to not only learn some new moves, but also get you out on the dance floor and meet new people. Latin Dance works your legs, buttocks, hips and waist and also improves your coordination and rhythm. After some practice, it can also really boost your self-esteem, especially if you find a great dance partner who meshes well with your particular style. Find a dance studio near you and ask about classes and outings.

Workout #1: Railings and Benches - The Best HIIT Tools

1. Warm up: Jumping Jacks for 1 minute
2. Jog for 1 minute
3. Sprint for 30 seconds

On a park bench:

4. 20 Single-leg Step Ups on each side
5. 20 Squat Jumps up onto the bench
6. 20 Triceps Dips: crouch down with your back facing away from the bench and place your hands on the end of the bench. Push yourself up and down, keeping your elbows in.
7. Jog for 1 minute
8. Sprint for 30 seconds

Railing

9. 20 Incline Pushups with your hands on the railing
10. 20 Plié Squat Jumps: Put your hands on the rail and stand with your feet together, facing outwards. Bend your knees slightly and jump out into a squat with your feet still facing out. Jump back in and repeat.
11. 10 Burpees
12. Jog for 1 minute
13. Sprint for 30 seconds

Rest for 2-3 minutes and repeat:
Beginner: 1 round
Intermediate: 2 rounds
Advanced: 3 rounds

Workout #2: Bodyweight HIIT

You can do this inside or take it outdoors.

1.   Warm up: Jump rope for 2 minutes
3.   Pushups: 20 times
3. Jumping Lunge: Starting in a lunge position, swing up your arms and jump in order to switch legs. You should land in a lunge position on the other side. Repeat 20 times.
4.   Chair or Bench Triceps Dips 10-15 times.
5.   Mountain Climber: In a pushup position, bend your right leg and move it up on the ground towards your chest while moving your left hand up as well. Move your body forward. Alternate hand and feet so you are moving forward. Take 30 steps. If you are outside do this on the grass.
5.   Crab Walk: Sit on the ground with your knees bent and feet on the ground and your hands behind you. Lift up your hips and tighten your abs as you move backwards. Take 30 steps.

Rest for 2 minutes and repeat once if you are a beginner, twice if you are intermediate, and three times if you are advanced.

Workout #3: HIIT the Court

This is the perfect HIIT workout to do on a basketball court at your gym or in the park.

1. Warm up: Do 50 jumping jacks at an easy pace
2. Sprints: Sprint from one end of the court to the other and jog back. Repeat 5 times.
3. Diagonal Hops: Standing on one side of the full court line, jump diagonally to the other side of the line. Then jump again to the other side so you are moving forward. Jump until you complete the length of the full-court line.
4. Sprints: Sprint from one side of the court to the other, and run backwards on the way back. Repeat 5 times.
5. Side Shuffles: Do side shuffles from one side of the court to the other. For added difficulty, keep your knees bent. When you reach the other side, side shuffle back. Repeat 2 times.
6. Jumping Jacks: 30 at an easy pace.

Rest for 2-3 minutes and repeat:
Beginner: 1 round
Intermediate: 2 rounds
Advanced: 3 rounds

Top.me

15 LOSE WEIGHT FROM SWIMMING

Swimming is an ideal low-impact cardiovascular workout that burns high calories, builds stamina and endurance and uses all the major muscles in your body (upper and lower). Swimming can be more intense than running, if the strokes are performed correctly and at the right intensity.

Swimming is a full body workout and the major muscles help power you through the water, helping with strength as well as calorie burning. It can be a fun activity to attend with friends or perfect for going alone and relaxing. It has been proven to help you unwind, relieve stress and even minimize symptoms of depression. It does not cost a lot to go swimming, as all you essentially need is a swimming costume/trunks, and possibly goggles and hat, plus the fee to a local swimming pool.

Swimming is gentle on your joints and perfect for people who have weak bones or are recovering from injury. Due to the buoyancy in the water, you can perform intense exercise without feeling pain ... although your muscles may feel it the following day!

There are many strokes to choose from when swimming, which helps keep it a varied exercise, and each stroke uses different muscles and has individual benefits. If you use a mixture of strokes, you are more likely to work the whole body and see more results, as well as balance your muscle groups.

Technique

It is crucial to master good swim strokes, form and technique, especially if you are a novice. It may be worth investing in a few lessons to refresh your memory or asking a swimming instructor or friend to watch you swim and help you improve your form. If your breathing technique or stroke is wrong, it can hinder your exercise regime and tire certain muscles out unnecessarily. If your muscles are fatigued early on, it can hinder your whole swimming session. Although swimming is easy on your joints and great for rehabilitation, it is strenuous exercise for your muscle groups.

Here are some of the most popular swimming strokes and their benefits:

Front Crawl / Freestyle

The front crawl is a fast stroke which focuses on your core. Good breathing technique is important for this stroke, as you need to swim close to the surface of the water with your head immersed, until you tilt to the side for breath. It involves kicking quickly to propel through the water and lifting your arms in and out of the water in fast strokes, with your body straight. A lot of the movement comes from your core muscles, which really benefits you if you get this technique correct. Front crawl is the most streamlined stroke for your body and helps your glide through the water quicker than others, causing less splash and more speed and lots of power from your hips. Front crawl will burn more calories than backstroke when swum at the same intensity. Whereas front crawl works your upper back and lats, breaststroke uses the pecs, so for a balance it is best to combine strokes.

Breaststroke

Breaststroke is a fairly gently stroke and an especially good choice for beginners. It works your whole body but is much slower and gentler than front crawl. If performed correctly, the breaststroke will work out your arm muscles (biceps and triceps), pectorals, shoulders, back, glutes and major leg muscles. To perform the stroke efficiently, you must perfect the breathing involved, which also improves lung capacity and helps you glide through the water better. Many women opt for breaststroke, especially for toning the 'difficult areas; such as the inner and outer thighs and glutes.

Butterfly

Of all the strikes, the butterfly is the best for burning calories and building muscles. It can burn up to 900 calories an hour. Although an hour of the butterfly stroke would be very heavy going and leave you incredibly sore the next day! Muscular power is needed to move your body in and out of the water in the butterfly stroke and it involves short, burst of power and movement to get you from one side to another. It is also one of the most difficult strokes to master and is vigorous on your body, which may lead to early fatigue, especially if you haven't mastered the technique properly.

back swimming

Backstroke

This can be a fast and easy stroke to master. Lying on your back, kick your legs and propel your arms. It is particularly useful for those who find underwater swimming and breathing difficult, as it does not involve putting your face into the water. It works the major muscles in your arms and legs, while strengthening your core muscles that help keep you flat along the water's surface.

For general cardio workouts, it is worthwhile introducing swimming into your routine, perhaps at a comfortable intensity for 2 or 3 times a week and 30-45 minute sessions. If you are working to improve your endurance and strength, introduce some interval training into your sessions (few minutes of very fast swimming, followed by slower minutes to recover), and incorporate some rest days. Although it may not feel like it at the time, swimming is a heavy workout for your body and muscles and you will need time to repair.

Swimming works well with other forms of exercise, as it is so different and can really mix up your regime and stop boredom setting in. Many people use swimming as a form of therapy, as it can be relaxing and ease symptoms such as stress and anxiety. Water has soothing and healing qualities and it's great for your wellbeing. The strokes allow you to stretch the muscles in your body without the impact and feelings you'd get if you were exercising on dry land, but you can still be safe in the knowledge that you are giving your body a great, all over workout.

16 JULY

Time to hit the beach to get that beach body! This month's High Intensity Interval Trainings are designed around the water. Even if you don't have a beach nearby you can use your local pool for most of the workouts.

The beauty of swimming is it is a very low-impact full body workout that not only tones your arms, back and legs, it also lets you cool off on those hot summer days. For these workouts, it is recommended you stock up on sunscreen.

For the swimming HIITs, it is recommended that you use swimming goggles and a swimming cap to keep your focus on your training.

Tip of the Month: Jogging on the Sand

If you have every jogged on the sand before, you will know it is quite the challenge. Your foot sinks into the sand and it is harder to get the impulse you have running on a treadmill or on a track when you lift your leg off the ground. However, it is this added challenge that makes running on the sand such a great workout. While it is tougher, and thus burns more calories, it is lower impact which makes it better for your knees. Keep in mind, however, that running in the sand may mean you run at a slower pace and you might get more tired faster. One tip is wearing shoes you don't mind getting wet and running closer to the water where the sand is more compacted. It makes it less laborious to run, but you still get many of the benefits of running in the sand. If you try this out, it is recommended you run in the morning or in the evening to prevent dehydration from the direct sun during the day.

Workout #1: Sand Hopping

1.   Warm up: Skipping. Avoid going into the parts closer to the water where the sand is compact. Skip down the sand trying to jump up as high and as far as you can jumping and landing on the same foot and alternating sides. Skip for 30 seconds.

2.   Squat Jump: Stand with your legs hip-width apart and put your hands behind your head or bent in front of you. Squat down as low as you can and jump up as high as you can. Land back down in squat position. Repeat 20 times.

3.   Single-leg Bounding: This workout is similar to skipping, but the switching is continuous. Bring up your right leg as your jump off your left leg and glide through the air. As soon as you hit the ground with your right leg, use your left leg's impulse to bring your right leg off the ground. Try to do this as high as far as you can for the maximum workout. Repeat for 20 switches.

4.   Side Lunge: Make three parallel lines in the sand about 4-5 yards apart. Straddle the middle line and shuffle to the right, bending your knees to touch the line. Life yourself up and shuffle to the farthest line. Repeat 20 times.

Rest for two minutes and repeat once if you are a beginner, twice if you are intermediate, and three times if you are advanced. Remember to stretch afterwards.

Workout #2: Freestyle swimming

As a warm up to HIIT swimming, take this simple but effective workout to the pool.

1.   Warm up: easy breast stroke for 5 minutes (2 x 25m laps)
2.   3 minute freestyle sprint (4 x 25m laps)
3.   4 minute easy breast stroke (4 x 25m laps)
4.   2 freestyle sprint (8 x 25m laps)
5.   4 minute easy breast (4 x 25m laps)
6.   3 minute freestyle sprint (10x 25m laps)
7.   8 minute easy freestyle (8 x 25m laps)

Rest for 5 minutes and repeat until your feel comfortable. If you are new to swimming, one cycle might be enough.

Workout #3: Swimming Ladder

1.   Warm up by jogging for 5-10 minutes on the sand or on the pavement near the pool.

2.   Get in the pool or water and swim an easy freestyle for 150 meters.

3.   Rest for 1 minute

4.   Freestyle 125 meters at a medium pace

5.   Rest for 1 minute

6.   Freestyle 100 meters at a sprint

7.   Rest for 1 minute

8.   Freestyle 125 meters at a medium pace

9.   Rest for 1 minute

10.   Freestyle 150 meters at a slow pace.

11.   Rest for one minute

12.   Cool down by holding the edge of the pool or resting your hands on the sand in a shallow area and kicking your legs, slowly bringing down the pace for about 3 minutes.

Depending on your conditioning, you might want to stop here or repeat the cycle 1-2 more times. Remember not to overwork yourself! After you are finished, stretch out.

Top.me

17 QUICK AND DELICIOUS GREEN SMOOTHIE RECIPES

Making a green smoothie daily for yourself and your family is one of the healthiest things you can do to start your day. They are delicious at any time of the day, but I have found that they make for the perfect breakfast. They are quick to make and will take you less overall time than cooking a traditional breakfast.

By green smoothie, I mean a smoothie that has both fruits and vegetables in it. Green smoothies are loaded with vitamins, nutrients, antioxidants, fiber. Ever since I have started making green smoothies for myself daily I have lost body fat, increased my energy levels and feel like my skin has improved.

No matter what your fitness goals are, green smoothies can help get you there. If you are trying to build lean muscle you can add in whey or soy protein powder. If you are looking to lose weight, green smoothies are great because they have high amounts of fiber that will help to keep you full longer.

Many people are scared off by anything "green." The key is in the combination of fruits and vegetables. There are some combinations of green smoothies that go much better together than others.

The three recipes that I am going to share below are great for someone who just started drinking green smoothies and is scared that they are going to taste too much like "vegetables."

The key to your green drinks tasting delicious is to use butter leaf lettuce, romaine lettuce, spinach, or kale as these blend deliciously with fresh fruit. If you are new to green drinks, you should start off with butter leaf or romaine lettuce and work your way up to kale and spinach leaves. Frozen fruits are also great for your green smoothies and give the drink an ice cream shake-like consistency. Frozen banana always blends deliciously and will mask the taste of the spinach and kale.

Kale is my favorite green ingredient because it is one of the healthiest and most nutrient-dense foods in the world. Kale scares a lot of people away because of its bitter taste but when combined with the right ingredients, you can hardly even taste it. I have found that my favorite green smoothies are the ones that contain kale and tropical fruits. Tropical fruits that blend deliciously with kale are mango, coconut, and pineapple. Orange juice makes for a great liquid base for smoothies.

If some of the smoothies taste too "bitter", swap romaine lettuce or butter leaf lettuce for kale and spinach. Get creative with your green smoothie recipes as you can even add ingredients such as avocado, carrot juice, or cauliflower.

Green Tropical Powerhouse

1 Cup Orange Juice
¼ Cup Frozen Mango
¼ Cup Frozen Banana
½ Cup Organic Spinach Leaves
½ Cup Greek Yogurt

Kale Colada

1 Cup Coconut Milk
½ Cup Frozen Pineapple
½ frozen Banana
½ Cup Kale Leaves

Green Strawberry and Bananas

1 1/2 Cup Orange Juice
¼ Cup Strawberry
1 Banana
¼ Cup Romaine Lettuce
¼ Cup Spinach leaves
¼ Cup Greek Yogurt

Tropical Green Paradise

1 ½ Cup Orange Juice
¼ Kiwi
¼ Cup Frozen Mango
¼ Cup Frozen Pinneapple
2 Tbsp Coconut Oil
¼ Cup Kale
¼ Cup Spinach

Green Antioxidant

1 Cup Pomegranate Juice
¼ Cup Kale Leaves
¼ Cup Blueberry
¼ Cup Raspberry
2 Tbsp Chia Seeds

Top.me

18 AUGUST

We are in the climax of the summer season and in our eighth month of HIIT. This month we work on legs, hips and core, which will help give you strength and confidence not only in workouts, but in daily activities.

We have also included a pure cardio workout, and we encourage you to take your runs outside rather than staying on the treadmill to take advantage of the summer warmth and get some fresh air.

Tip of the Month: Berry Smoothie

Most berries are in season and making smoothies are a great way to stay hydrated as well as to get your daily dose of antioxidants and vitamins. Try this smoothie as a pre or post workout snack.

- 1 cup fresh mixed berries
- 1 frozen banana
- ½ cup low-fat vanilla yogurt
- 1 tbsp. protein powder (vanilla)
- ¼ cup orange juice

Put all of the ingredients in a blender and enjoy!

Workout #1:

1.   Squat Rear Lunge: Stand straight with feet a little wider tan hip-width apart and your hands behind your head. Come down to a full squat and take one leg back so you are in a lunge. Pulse for 2 seconds, and come back into a squat. Stand up, keeping your back straight and abs firm, and switch legs. Repeat 10 times each side.

2.   Jump Squat: Start in a squat position with your legs together. Jump up as high as you can and land in a squat position with your legs apart. Continue as fast as you can without losing form for 1 minute

3.   Squat Plank Push-up: Start in a squat with your hands on the ground and jump into plank position with legs hip-width apart. Go down into a pushup and back up into a plank. Jump your feet back into a squat. Complete 15.

4.   Jump Squat

5.   Side to Side Lunges: Stand with your feet together and your hands on your hips. Come down to your left side into a side lunge without let your bent knee past your foot. Come up again and step your feet together. Stop to the other side. Repeat 10 times each side, or 15 times if you are advanced

6.   Jump Squat

Rest for two minutes and repeat the cycle 2 times if you are beginner, 3 if you are intermediate, and 4 if you are advanced.

Workout #2: Abs Power

You can do this work out in a park or in your neighborhood.

1. Warm up: Jog for 2 minutes
2. Knee Highs: Run bringing your knees up towards your chest for 2 minutes
3. Butt Kickers: Run bringing your feet to your buttocks for 2 minutes
4. Plank Pipe Jumps: Start in plank position and hold for 10 seconds, jump your feet towards your hands, finishing in a low squat. Jump again, pulling your legs back into a plank. Repeat 5 times.
5. V Sit-ups: Lie down on the grass or ground facing up with your hands behind your head. Bring up your knees, legs together towards your upper body as your upper body moves towards your legs. Repeat 20 times
6. Plank Jumping Jacks : Start in a plank position on your forearms with your feet together. Jump and separate your legs until they form a Y with your body. Jump your feet together and repeat up to 20 times. Make sure to keep your core firm and in a straight line with your neck and hips.
7. Tabletop Dip: Sit down on the grass or ground with your knees bent towards the ceiling. Put your hands on the floor behind your back. Balance on your heels. Push your middle body up into a table top, stretching out your arms. Repeat 20 times

Rest for 2-3 minutes and repeat:
Beginner: 1 round
Intermediate: 2 rounds
Advanced: 3 rounds

Workout #3:

This simple sprinting and jogging workout can be combined with or switched off with the strength building HIITs in this month's guide. Remember to finish off with some good stretching to prevent injuries.

1. Warm up: Jog for 5 minutes
2. Sprint: 100 yards or 15 seconds
3. Jog 1 minute
4. Sprint 125 yards or 20 seconds
5. Jog 1 minute
6. Sprint 100 yards or 15 seconds
7. Jog 1 minute
8. Sprint 125 yards or 20 seconds
9. Jog 1 minute

Rest for 2-3 minutes and repeat:
Beginner: 1 round
Intermediate: 2 rounds
Advanced: 3 rounds

19 SIX REASONS YOU SHOULD DRINK MORE WATER AND 10 TIPS TO ACTUALLY DO IT

Many of us drink water because we know we should, few people actually understand the benefits of drinking water. From keeping us awake to making sure our muscles work properly, there are tons of unexpected benefits. Here are the most surprising reasons you should be drinking more water every day.

Water is Muscle Fuel

When you exercise, you sweat in order to help your body regulate its temperature. Some of this water comes directly from your muscles, and as your muscles dehydrate, they also get tired much quicker. If you aren't constantly replenishing your muscles with fluids, not only will your routine get cut short, but you will also feel pretty bad. Sport drinks, which do a great job of making you think it is what your body is craving for when you exercise, aren't necessarily the best thing to be drinking as a regular hydration regimen because of the large amounts of sugar they contain. However, if you are already very dehydrated or low on energy, studies performed at the Department of Gastroenterology of the University Hospital, Maastricht, The Netherlands[12], show these drinks can be effective with regards to glucose (energy) absorption. Before reaching for the fruity, sugary drinks, try downing a bottle of water and your muscles should pick up in no time.

Water Can Help Fight Acne

---

[12]M. A. Van Nieuwenhoven, R.-J. M. Brummer, F. Brouns (2000), Gastrointestinal function during exercise: comparison of water, sports drink, and sports drink with caffeine, Journal of Applied Physiology,89(3): 1079-1085

Toxins and bacteria that circulate the body and deposit in the skin can clog your pores, and can cause inflammation and acne. One of waters functions is to flush out toxins from your body, which can reduce the amount of bacterial toxins that cause reactions in your skin. When you are dehydrated, toxins and bacteria stay in the skin causing your skin to react by inflaming around the infection. However, if you drink lots of water and eat healthy, your skin has an easier time maintaining a hydration balance and your body can more easily flush out harmful acne-causing toxins.

Water Optimizes Kidney Function

Your kidneys are the organs responsible for regulating the level of electrolytes in your body, maintaining a healthy blood pressure, and serve as a filter for the blood, eliminating any and all unwanted materials and reabsorbing those that are useful for the body. All of this depends on the level of water homeostasis, or fluid intake and water balance in the body. Not drinking enough water can result in urinary tract infections and renal stones, two very painful illnesses, your better off avoiding. You can help to avoid renal failure, and help the body to filter toxins simply by drinking enough water a day!

Water Can Replace Your Coffee

One of the most common symptoms of dehydration is tiredness and fatigue, which in many settings can lead us to reach for the coffee pot. Unfortunately, coffee is a diuretic, meaning it will actually lead to increased fluid loss. Drinking lots of water will help ease the tiredness caused by dehydration, not to mention, getting up more often to go to the bathroom will keep you on your toes.

Water Can Keep You "Regular"

Constipation can be caused by a range of factors, including lack of exercise and low fiber and fluid intake. Before hitting the drug store to see what drugs can help the "flow", you might want to try hydrating first. Fluid intake helps to ease the passage of stool through the colon, making you feel better and keeping your intestines healthy. Studies by the Nestlé Water Institute, Vittel, France[13], show that even when laxatives are taken to ease constipation, there is a reduction in efficacy if the patient is not well hydrated.

Water Can Boost Brain Function

While short-term changes in cognitive function are often attributed to nutrition, we shouldn't overlook the importance of water intake with regards to a healthy brain function. A study carried out with children[14] showed that even a 1-2% reduction in body weight loss due to fluid loss can significantly impair cognitive function. Drinking enough water can help keep you more alert, and even improve your mood, keeping your brain happy and functioning well.

Bonus: Exactly How Much Water Should You Be Drinking?

While the 8-8oz glasses a day is used as a benchmark, the amount of water you actually need depends on your weight, level of exercise, and the amount of alcoholic and caffeinated drinks you consume a day. Here is how you can calculate how much water you should be drinking a day:

Divide your weight in two. This tells you how many ounces of water you should be drinking a day, assuming you lead a sedentary lifestyle and do not drink alcoholic or caffeinated beverages

Add 8oz to that base amount for every 15 minutes of

---

[13] http://www.nature.com/ejcn/journal/v57/n2s/full/1601907a.html

[14] D'Anci, K. E., Constant, F. and Rosenberg, I. H. (2006), Hydration and Cognitive Function in Children. Nutrition Reviews, 64: 457–464.

exercise you do a day

Add 8oz for every cup you drink of an alcoholic or caffeinated beverage

For example, if I weigh 150 lbs, I exercise 1 hour a day, and I drink 1 cola a day, I should be drinking:

$(150/2) + 8 + 16 = 99oz$ or 12 glasses of water a day.

Remember that we can only survive a few days without water, which highlights the importance of fluid intake every day. Remember that fruits and vegetables also contain a high water content, so it is a great alternative if you aren't a fan of good old H2O.

How Much Water Is Too Much Water?

Technically, yes, you can drink too much water, but it is very rare. If you are a generally healthy person, it is very difficult to overhydrate. People with chronic health diseases like renal failure or heart disease, sometimes have a harder time processing foods and liquids in general, so the extra stress on the body of having to process excess amounts of water in order to keep the mineral balance of the blood can be too much for your body. However, unless your doctor indicates that you have to watch your water intake, which is very unusual, you shouldn't have to worry about drinking too much water.

How to Remind Yourself to Drink Water

There is a great trick you can use to remind yourself to drink enough water. After you figure out how much you should be drinking using the formula above, get a large water bottle or use two normal-sized ones. Take a permanent water and mark your goal to drink an inch and a half every hour or so, until your quota of water is done and the day is over. If you get used to drinking small amounts throughout the day, rather than lots of water all at once, you're bound to drink more and stay hydrated more consistently. Soon, you'll find that your body is still craving water even after meeting your goal

10 Tips to Drink More Water

Some people refrain from drinking as much water as they should simply because they don't like the taste of it, or it's simply too boring to be drinking so much all day. There are some simple tips you can follow to keep your water drinking interesting and even give it some extra nutrients.

Add a Lemon or Lime Slice

Adding little bit of citrus can make all of the difference when your tastes buds need some stimulation in what you drink. You can add half a lemon cut in slices in your water pitcher or water bottle overnight and drink first think in the morning or throughout your day to stimulate your immune system.

Infuse With Fruit

Add some of your favorite berries to your water and lightly mash with a fork to squeeze out the flavor. It also gives the water a great color, which can stimulate your appetite.

Pick Your Favorite Fruit and Add a Bit of Stevia

Using some of the tips above may not be enough, especially if your taste buds are used to drinking sweet juices or sodas. Stevia is a great alternative to cane sugar, since it is actually sweeter but it has no calories, and best of all, it is derived from a plant. It comes in powder or liquid form, and both taste equally yummy.

Add Low-calorie Flavor Powder Packs

There are tons of flavor and brand alternatives out there these days, and many of them come in handy one-serving packets that you can pour in your water bottle and shake.

Use a Straw

It may seem like such a silly tip, but you will be surprised at how much more water your drink! It makes it easier for you to take smaller sips at smaller intervals, and it also helps keep you from swallowing air, as can happen when taking big gulps.

Find Out How You Like Your Water

You might be thinking, "wait, water is not coffee!" However, each person, depending on their mood and time of day, prefer drinking their water ice cold, cool, or room temperature. If you are a person who is more sensitive to cold, it may even be painful for you to drink very cold water. For others, drinking water at room temperature can make them feel sick. So, try different alternatives, and see which one is most pleasant to you.

Eat More Fruits And Vegetables

Most fruits and vegetables have a very high water content. Celery, for example is 95% water, and apples are 84% water. Not only do fruits and veggies give your body tons of the vitamins, nutrients, and fiber you need, they also help to keep you hydrated.

Try Sparkling Water

Sparkling water has no calories, sugar or artificial flavoring, but it gives you the same sensation in your mouth as if you were drinking soda. You can mash up some berries at the bottom of you glass and add sparking water to spruce it up a bit.

Add a Splash of Juice or Fruit Syrup

Even better if the juice is unsweetened, adding very little

juice can give your water the flavor you need to gulp it down and hydrate.

Add Mint Leaves

If you let the mint soak enough, it infuses the water with the taste of iced mint tea. You can squeeze lemon juice right in if you feel it needs more of a kick.

Top.me

20 SEPTEMBER

Summer is just about over but the weather is still mild enough to take some of our workouts outside. We are three-quarters through the year and you should be feeling good about your strength, resistance and tone thanks to all of the HIIT you have been doing these past months. Don't let the rhythm fall now!

Tip of the Month: Add Music to Your Workout

Listening to music as you work out can actually boost the exercise effectiveness, particularly for those who practice high intensity interval training. It can make a workout feel easier and less monotonous, and will help you keep up the tempo, burning more calories in a shorter amount of time. Do you have your workout playlist yet?

Workout 1: Buns of Steel

1.   Warm-up with a jump rope for 30 seconds.

2.   Deadlift Balance: Start standing straight with your hand behind you head and your left foot slightly behind your hips on your toes. Shift forward until your upper body is parallel with the ground, keeping your upper body and back leg into a straight line. Shift back to your starting position. Repeat on the same side 10 times and shift legs.

3.   Side-to-side Shuffle Jump: Stand straight with your feet a little wider than hip width apart. Come down into a squat and touch the ground next to your right foot and as you come back up again jump as high as you can. Come back into a squat and touch the ground next to the other foot, jumping as you come back up. Repeat 10 times each side.

4.   Jump Rope for 2 minutes

5.   Lunge Kicks: From full lunge position, push yourself up with your back leg and use the momentum from that same leg to kick up as high as you can. Lower back down into lunge position. Do 20 on each side.

Rest for two minutes and repeat the cycle 2 times if you are beginner, 3 if you are intermediate, and 4 if you are advanced.

Workout #2: Washboard Abs

1.   Jumping Jacks: for 2 minutes
2.   Bicycle Crunches: for 45 seconds
3.   Flutter Kicks: Lie down on the ground and place your hands under your buttocks, palms down. Hover both feet off of the ground, close together. Lift one foot up about three-4 feet of the ground and switch legs. Continue for 45 seconds.
4.   Jumping Jacks: for 2 minutes.
5.   Russian Twists: Start in a contracted crunch position. Clasp your hands together in front of you, elbows out. Twist to one side of your body, than the other. Continue for 45 seconds.
6.   Toe Touches: Lying on the ground, lift your legs up so that they are at a 90° angle with the floor. With your arms straight up, lift your torso so your hands touch your feet, or as close to them as possible. Bring your back down to the floor.
7.   Jumping Jacks for 2 minutes

Rest for 3 minutes. Beginners repeat once, intermediate repeat twice and advanced repeat 3 times.

Workout #3: Legs and Abs

1. Jump Rope: for 2 minutes
2. Hip Bridge: Lie on your back and your legs bent so your feet are flat on the ground, about hip-width apart. Place your arms at your sides, palms down. Lift your hips until you form a straight line from your knees to your shoulders, contracting your glutes and your back. Bring your hips slowly down again. Repeat 20 times.
3. Jump Rope for 2 minutes
4. Plank Toe Touch: Start in plank position with your forearms on the ground and feet together. While keeping your right leg straight, move it off to the side about 2 feet and tap your toe on the ground. Move it back to center and to the same with the opposite leg. Repeat 20 times.
5. Jump Rope for 2 minutes
6. V-ups: Lie on the ground with your legs straight and your arms stretched over your head. Keep your legs straight and your arms in line with your upper body, and bring your legs and upper body off the ground so it forms a "V". Repeat 20 times.
7. Jump Rope for 2 minutes

Rest for 2-3 minutes and repeat:
Beginner: 1 round
Intermediate: 2 rounds
Advanced: 3 rounds

21 OCTOBER

Fall is here! The leaves are turning and the hoodies are coming out for our workouts. Don't let the weather transition get you down. This month, we will be taking out High Intensity Interval Training back inside with the elliptical machine, resistance bands and more. Remember that as the weather cools down, the best way to stay warm is to get your heart pumping.

Tip of the Month: Pumpkins as a Workout Tool

Before you start carving your pumpkins for the Halloween festivities, use them as weights! They come in all shapes and sizes and you can use the larger ones in the same way as you would a medicine ball. The smaller ones you can use as free weights for some moves. Try mixing some pumpkins into your abdominal training with moves like Russian twists and sit-ups. You can also work biceps, triceps and shoulders by using smaller pumpkins instead of free weights. Try some of the following exercises with pumpkins!

Workout #1: Warming Up to the Elliptical

Not all elliptical machines are made alike, which is why it is hard to give instructions in terms of force or speed. In the following exercises, the "work" phase is where you are at your maximum effort. The rest phase is more leisurely and that is the time you should use to recover.

1. Warm up: a moderate pace for 5 minutes. Explore a comfortable resistance level and ramp height.
2. Work: maximum effort for 30 seconds
3. Rest: moderate pace for 2 minutes
4. Work: maximum effort for 30 seconds
5. Rest: moderate pace for 1 minute 30 seconds
6. Work: maximum effort for 30 seconds
7. Rest: moderate pace for 1 minute
8. Work: maximum effort for 30 seconds
9. Rest: moderate pace for 1 minute 30 seconds
10. Work: maximum effort for 30 seconds
11. Rest: moderate pace for 2 minutes

Rest for 2-3 minutes and repeat:
Beginner: 1 round
Intermediate: 2 rounds
Advanced: 3 rounds

Workout #2: Front-Back Elliptical Routine

1. 3 minutes warm-up at resistance 0
2. 3 minutes at resistance 4
3. 2 minutes at resistance 6
4. 2 minutes backwards, at resistance 3
5. 3 minutes at resistance 10
6. 2 minutes at resistance 8
7. 1 minute at resistance 11
8. 3 minutes backwards at resistance 10
9. 3 minutes at resistance 8
10. 3 minutes at resistance 6

11. 2 minutes backwards at resistance 6
12. 3 minutes at resistance 3

Unless you are looking for a big challenge, there is no need to repeat this exercise. If you are less experienced, bring down the effort and if you are advanced, step it up.

Workout #3: Resistance Band

You can try some of these with pumpkins instead of resistance bands!

1.   Warm up on the elliptical machine at a moderate pace for 5 minutes

2.   Leg Extensions: Place the legs of the chair over the resistance band and sit on the chain. Slip your feet through each handle. Extend your legs outwards one at a time, holding onto the sides of the chair for balance. Repeat 20 times.

3.   Thigh Squeeze: Start in the same position as above, but extend your legs straight outward. Open your legs in a V and bring back together. Repeat 20 times.

4.   Elliptical at max effort for 3 minutes, then at a moderate pace for 2 minutes

5.   Biceps Curls: Stand on a resistance band and hold the handles in each hand. Keep your elbows close to your body and bring your hands towards your shoulders. Repeat 20 times.

6.   Shoulder Press: Stand on the resistance band and hold the handles in each hand. Bring the band on the outer part of each bent arm. Bring up your elbows up to shoulder level, and back down at your sides again. Repeat 20 times.

7.   Elliptical at max effort for 3 minutes, then at a moderate pace for 2 minutes

8.   Cool down for 3 additional minutes on the elliptical

If you are at a good energy level, repeat the cycle.

22 FOUR EASY WAYS TO BOOST YOUR FITNESS MOTIVATION

Let's face it- working out consistently can be hard. Getting back into the workout rhythm after summer is a challenge. It is so unfair – after a short break, like a summer vacation, starting to work out again feels like starting from scratch!

On days when we are lacking motivation and are tired chances are we are not going to work out. The problem with this approach and mindset is these kinds of decisions are habit forming and you will continue to make up excuses in your head to not workout.

So what are the best ways to get motivated about your Fitness and workout more regularly? Let's take a look at a few things you can start doing right away to boost your motivation.

New Music Play List

Something as simple as a new music play list can really amp up your motivation and your workout. On days when you are physically tired, try listening to a new set of music that really excites you. This will distract your mind temporarily and you

119

will be focusing on the enjoyment of the music instead of the physical pain of the workout. I have found that my best workouts occur when I have a new music play list.

Set Short Term Goals to Reach Long Term Objectives

This may sound confusing but is a really great goal setting process. Maybe your long term fitness goal is to look like a certain celebrity or lose a certain number of lbs. If the goal is realistically more than a few months away, it is important to stay on track and not lose focus of the small baby steps you have to consistently take to get there. The problem with a goal so far away is people are impatient and lose track of the main objective. You should set a fitness objective for every 2 weeks that will help you reach your long-term fitness goal. Focus on meeting your two-week goal every time and before you know it you will be at your long term goal.

New Fitness Wardrobe

Let's be honest – it is fun to train in the newest and best training shoes and training gear. Sometimes picking out some new and exciting fitness clothes can get you to the gym and get you jumpstarted again. I know when I get a new pair of training shoes or new gym outfits I am more excited to work out that day. It is fun to change up your usual fitness look and routine.

Visual Inspiration

When it comes to fitness, the best motivation is definitely visual. When you have a visual representation of what you want to look like it will drive you to train a lot harder and more consistently. We all want to look our best and need a little visual motivation once in a while.

Take your Workout Outside

Sometimes the best thing you can do to boost your

motivation is to change up the scenery of your workouts. If you are constantly training in a dark gym it can become mundane and depressing.

In October, it's still warm enough to go outside to train. There are many great workouts you can do with minimal or no equipment.

Top.me

23 NOVEMBER

We're in the home stretch! The year is winding down and things tend to get busier, making it harder to find time to work out. However, as the holiday season approaches, it's important to stay on top of your daily HIIT so you keep from gaining back the weight you've worked so hard to lose this year.

This month, we have shorter, more intense HIITs to get the most out of your workout without it cutting into your end-of the year schedule too much.

Tip of the Month: Leaf Obstacle Course

The trees will lose most of their leaves this month, covering your lawns, yards, sidewalks, and driveways. The job has to be done, so we might as well make a it a workout! Before you bag the leaves, make an obstacle course by making large leaf piles one after another that you can jump over. Make smaller piles or lines to run around. If you want to make a party out of it, make different activities that include finding a ball in a leaf pile, rolling through leaves, making something with them, and finally who can rake them up fastest. Involve the kids, you'll have a blast, beat the stress, and get your daily workout in!

Workout #1:

1. Warm up: Jumping Jacks for 1 minute
2. Jumping Jacks For 1 minute
3. Alternating Toe Touch: Stand straight with your legs hip-width apart bring your left leg straight up in a controlled manner and try to touch it with your right hand. Switch. Continue for 30 seconds.
4. Butt Kickers: Run in place bringing your feet as close to your buttocks as you can, lightly kicking it with each foot, if possible. Make sure to keep up the energy.
5. Squat Jump: Start in a squat position with your hands bend together in front of you. Jump up, propelling yourself up as high as possible, and land in squat position again. Continue for 1 minute. Rest for 10 seconds.
6. Pushup Burpees: Start standing with your legs hip-width apart and crouch down with your hands on the floor in front of you. Jump your legs back until you are in a pushup position, go down into the push-up, and quickly jump your legs back under your body. Stand up again with your arms at your side. Continue for 1 minute Rest for 10 seconds.
7. Squat Jump. Rest for 10 seconds.
8. Pushup Burpees. Rest for 10 seconds.
9. Jog in Place

Repeat, if desired.

Workout #2:

Grab some 5-15lb dumbbells for this HIIT.

1.   Warm up: Jumping Jacks for 2 minutes.

2.   Standing Crisscross Crunches: Stand up straight with your legs hip-width apart and your hands behind your head. Bring up your left leg and cross your elbow trying to touch the top of your knee. Switch sides. Repeat for 30 seconds

3.   Jumping Jacks for 1 minute

4.   Knee up and outs: Still standing, bring your left knee straight up and down, then off to the side and down and straight forward and down. Switch sides. Repeat for 30 seconds.

5.   Lunge Overhead Press: Step your left leg back into lunge position. Hold one dumbbell in each hand. Hold the lunge position and perform overhead presses for 30 seconds.

6.   Jumping Jack Planks: In extended-arm plank position, keep your feet together. Jump your feet apart and then back together. Continue for 30 seconds.

7.   Triceps Bridges: Lie down on the ground with your knees bent. Lift up your hips but keep your shoulders on the ground. There should be a straight line from your knees to your shoulders. Hold one dumbbell in each hand. Stretch your arms over your head. Keep your arms straight, and while staying in the bridge position, lift your arms straight up, then onto the ground again.

8.   Jumping Jacks for 1 minute

Repeat, if desired.

Workout #3

You'll need a jump rope for the warm up and cool down.

1.   Start by jogging in place for 1 minute
2.   Jump Rope for 1 minute
3.   Burpees (without the pushup) for 30 seconds
4.   Pushups for 30 seconds
5.   Mountain Climbers for 30 seconds
6.   Side-crunch Plank for 30 seconds
7.   Toe Touch Crunches: Lie down on the ground and stretch your legs straight up into the air. Stretch your arms straight out and lift your upper body trying to touch your legs. Continue for 30 seconds.
8.   Jump Rope for 3 minutes

Repeat once if you are a beginner, twice if you are intermediate, and three times if you are advanced.

24 SIX SIMPLE TIPS TO STAY HEALTHY DURING THE HOLIDAYS

Ah, the holidays are coming. With all of the big family meals, delicious sweets, and plenty of specialty drinks to welcome the New Year, it's hard to even imagine it's possible to keep your diet. Here are a few tips to keep your healthy rhythm going without missing out on the fun.

Take Walks Before and After Meals

A lot of the time, the meals we eat for the holidays aren't necessarily unhealthy, but we eat such huge portions that we slowly pack on the pounds we tried so hard to lose the rest of the year. Taking walks before and after big meals will help you lose some of the calories you are about to consume, and taking a breath of fresh air will also help you relieve some of the stress.

Focus on the Fun, Not the Food

You may love your aunt's pumpkin pie, but try to keep your excitement focused on the family time and the opportunity to catch up with friends. Staying focused on people instead of food will have you eating less and building relationships more. Taking advantage of these moments will last much longer than that last bite of gingerbread! I know this is not an easy task, and it takes some mental preparation beforehand, but the practice will keep you in the moment and satisfied by the company, not the full belly.

Stop Eating Before You Feel Stuffed

When relatives visit and everyone brings something to share, it is easy to get overwhelmed and excited by all of the delicious holiday treats. The problem is, most of these foods tend to be high in refined sugar and saturated fats that are the culprit of quick weight gain and long-term health problems. One of the tricks is to eat slowly, really enjoy the food, and stop eating before you get to the point where you have to subtly unbutton your pants. Eat until you are satisfied, but don't go overboard. It takes up to twenty minutes for our brain to register when we are full, so eat slowly and make a conscious check about how hungry you still are before you serve yourself another piece of smoked ham.

Eat a Light, Healthy Meal Before Leaving the House

When we know we are going to have a big meal later on in the day, we often avoid eating at all to make sure we "make room" for the meal that is to come. However, skipping meals can cause overeating later on in the day, meaning in one sitting you may eat more than a day's worth of calories!

If you make up a fresh salad or munch on a red apple with a glass of water before you leave the house, you won't be starving by the time you get there. This way you can enjoy yourself without stuffing yourself.

Replace Unhealthy Ingredients for Healthier Ones

Take a look at your family recipes and pick out some of the more unhealthy ingredients. If a recipe calls for lard or bacon grease, switch it out for olive oil in smaller quantities. If it calls for large amounts of sugar, see if you can switch it out for stevia, a plant-based, no-calorie sweetener. Use skim milk or almond milk instead of whole milk.

These tips, used repeatedly in all of your favorite holiday

dishes will help limit your saturated fat and caloric intake, and in most cases no one will even know the difference!

Pick and Choose the Most Special Holiday Treats

We all know what our favorite dishes are during the holidays, but along the way we cannot help but try new things—sometimes more than once. Make your mantra "quality over quantity", and savor every piece of your favorite holiday dishes. When you are at a holiday party and get overwhelmed by all that there is to offer, just think about the treats you are really looking forward to and stick to those.

These tips have all been about your physical health during the holidays, but there is another aspect to consider. Always remember that your mental health is just as important as your physical health, so as the stress piles up while you think about everything you need to get done, make sure to take some time for yourself. Treat yourself to a massage or take time to watch your favorite movie. Making sure you avoid stress will also help you to avoid stress-eating. The best part of all? You'll feel so good in the new year when you realize that you have stayed on track, even through the holidays!

Top.me

25 DECEMBER

Congratulations! You made it through the year and hopefully you kept up exercising. Whether you are finally resting or working harder than ever during the holiday season, it is important that you keep up your workouts if you want to feel energetic and strong for the end of the year gatherings.

Tip of the Month: Snowball Fights

One way to keep active while enjoying the season is by going out and playing in the snow! No matter what your age, it is a great way to spend time with friends and family. Divide up into teams and see who can build the best snow fort. You can even play snowball freeze tag by deciding on boundaries, and having a team member from each side in charge of "tagging" the other team by hitting them with a snowball. When someone gets hit, they freeze and they can only be unfrozen when their team member touches them. The first team to freeze the entire other team wins. You'll get quite the cardio workout and not to mention have lots of laughs!

Workout #1: Stationary Bike Interval Training

1. 5 minutes of low intensity
2. 30 seconds high intensity at 70-75% maximum effort
3. 1 minute of low intensity.
4. 30 seconds high intensity at 80-85% maximum effort
5.   1 minute of low intensity.
6. 30 seconds high intensity at 90%+ maximum effort
7. 1 minute of low intensity.
8. 30 seconds high intensity at 90%+ maximum effort
9. 1 minute of low intensity.
10. 30 seconds high intensity at 80-85%+ maximum effort
11. 1 minute of low intensity.
12. 30 seconds high intensity at 80-85%+ maximum effort
13. 1 minute of low intensity.
14. 30 seconds high intensity at 70-75%+ maximum effort
15. 1 minute of low intensity.
16. 5 minutes of very low intensity to cool down.

Rest for 3 minutes and repeat once if you are a beginner, 2 times if you are intermediate, and 3 times if you are advanced.

Workout #2

1.   Forward Squat Jumps: Squat jump forward and then jump backwards landing in a squat. Repeat for 30 seconds.

2.   Sprint on the Spot: Run in place bringing your knees high to your chest as fast as you can, pumping your arms at the same time. 30 seconds.

3.   Alternating Plank: Start in plank position and step out one leg, then bring it back in. Then do the same with the other leg and repeat. Continue for 30 seconds.

4.   Regular Squat Jumps for 30 seconds.

5.   Sprint on the spot for 1 minute.

6.   Plan with Foot Raised: 15 seconds each side.

7.   Jumping Jacks: 1 minute.

8.   Plank with arm extension: In regular plank position, put one arm out overhead. Alternate after 15 seconds.

9.   Sprint on the spot for 30 seconds.

10.   Jumping Jacks for 1 minute.

11.   Sprints on the spot: three times 30 seconds, resting 15 seconds between each sprint.

Workout #3: Boxing Off the Calories

1. Warm up: each trotting with your jump rope, warm up at 20% intensity for 2 minutes

2. Jump Rope: Pick up to a 90% intensity for 1 minute

3. Recovery: Bring it back down to 20% for 1 minute

4. 50 straights: While one person is on the receiving end of the punches, the other punches 50 straights, alternating arms, back to back, as fast as you can. The one who is receiving should stand strong with arms firm and abs tucked in. Switch off.

5. Bicycle Crunches: 1 set of 20 crunches.

6. 50 uppercuts: Same as the first boxing set, the person on the receiving end should hold good posture and on the punching end complete them as fast as you can. Switch off.

7. Lunges: Do 15 lunges on each side.

8. 50 hooks: same as a above, and switch off.

9. Push-ups: carry out 15 push-us.

10. Straight, uppercut, hooks: do 10 of each, three cycles, and switch off.

11. Cool down: 2 min of jump rope at 20%

GOOD LUCK AND TO YOUR HEALTH

That is it from me! I hope you are having a healthy year. If you follow the plans in this book, or at least take some inspiration from them, you will have a starting point on your journey to be in shape, strong, and healthy.

From here on out, it is up to you to do the work to make the dream a reality (yes, you actually have to do some work).

Just remember to never let go of the dream and keep working every day towards your goal.

To your health!
Natalia Krasnyanskaya
& the team at www.top.me

ABOUT THE AUTHOR

Natalia Krasnyanskaya is the Editor in Chief of Top.me, the health & fitness site.

Covering the lifestyle, beauty, fashion, and health beats, she is an avid fitness enthusiast herself. She practices sports ranging from weight lifting to running, and even pole fitness.

Born and raised in eastern Ukraine, Natalia made her Master of Linguistics and Foreign Language at the Kharkov National University.

Natalia's motto is: Push Yourself - Nobody Is Going to Do It for You.

You can contact her personally any time at natalia@top.me.